Aesthetic Surgery

Current Perspectives

Concise Book for Bariatric and Cosmetic Surgery

Contributors

Ruchi Goel MS, DNB, FICS
Professor of Ophthalmology
Guru Nanak Eye Centre
Maulana Azad Medical College
New Delhi

Pavitra Ganguly MS
Professor of Surgery
Jamia Hamdard University
New Delhi

Neelima Gupta MS
Associate Professor of ENT
University College of Medical Sciences
New Delhi

Smriti Nagpal
Guru Nanak Eye Centre
New Delhi

Aesthetic Surgery

Current Perspectives

Concise Book for Bariatric and Cosmetic Surgery

Amit Goel

MS (Surgery), FICS, FNB (Minimal Access Surgery)

Associate Professor, General Surgery
Jamia Hamdard University, New Delhi, India
e-mail: *gamit11@rediffmail.com*

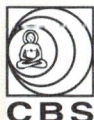

CBS Publishers & Distributors Pvt Ltd

New Delhi • Bengaluru • Chennai • Kochi • Mumbai • Pune
Hyderabad • Kolkata • Nagpur • Patna • Vijayawada

Aesthetic Surgery
Current Perspectives

ISBN: 978-81-239-2497-7

Copyright © Author and Publisher

First Edition: 2015

Published by Satish Kumar Jain for

CBS Publishers & Distributors Pvt Ltd

4819/XI Prahlad Street, 24 Ansari Road, Daryaganj, New Delhi 110 002, India.
Ph: 23289259, 23266861, 23266867   Website: www.cbspd.com
Fax: 011-23243014   e-mail: delhi@cbspd.com; cbspubs@airtelmail.in.
Corporate Office: 204 FIE, Industrial Area, Patparganj, Delhi 110 092
Ph: 4934 4934   Fax: 4934 4935   e-mail: publishing@cbspd.com; publicity@cbspd.com

Branches

- **Bengaluru:** Seema House 2975, 17th Cross, K.R. Road,
  Banasankari 2nd Stage, Bengaluru 560 070, Karnataka
  Ph: +91-80-26771678/79   Fax: +91-80-26771680   e-mail: bangalore@cbspd.com
- **Chennai:** 20, West Park Road, Shenoy Nagar, Chennai 600 030, Tamil Nadu
  Ph: +91-44-26260666, 26208620   Fax: +91-44-42032115   e-mail: chennai@cbspd.com
- **Kochi:** 36/14 Kalluvilakam, Lissie Hospital Road, Kochi 682 018, Kerala
  Ph: +91-484-4059061-65   Fax: +91-484-4059065   e-mail: kochi@cbspd.com
- **Mumbai:** 83-C, Dr E Moses Road, Worli, Mumbai-400018, Maharashtra
  Ph: +91-22-24902340/41   Fax: +91-22-24902342   e-mail: mumbai@cbspd.com
- **Pune:** Bhuruk Prestige, Sr. No. 52/12/2+1+3/2 Narhe, Haveli
  (Near Katraj-Dehu Road Bypass), Pune 411 041, Maharashtra
  Ph: +91-20-64704058/59, 32392277   Fax: +91-20-24300160   e-mail: pune@cbspd.com

Representatives

- **Hyderabad**   0-9885175004
- **Nagpur**   0-9021734563
- **Vijayawada**   0-9000660880
- **Kolkata**   0-9831437309, 0-9051152362
- **Patna**   0-9334159340

Printed at: HT Media Ltd., Noida

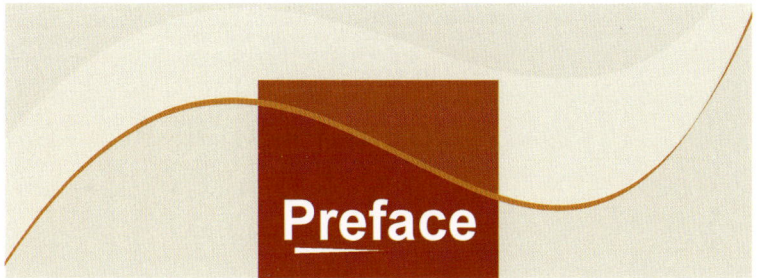
Preface

This book is a short synopsis on the current aspects of aesthetic surgery. It covers various topics of aesthetic surgery with focus on facial surgery.

Various aspects of morbid obesity, a major health concern in developing nations which doubled in the past 25 years, have also been discussed. Recent statistics indicate that obesity has reached epidemic proportions and that 700 million people would become obese by 2015. According to Economic Survey 2012, incidence of obesity is 26.1% in the UK and 36.5% in the USA. Bariatric surgery is the only effective treatment for morbid obesity.

The book elaborates the various aspects of maxillofacial surgery including rhinoplasty, face lift and eyelid cosmetic surgery. This book is meant for surgeons interested in various aspects of aesthetic surgery.

I express my gratitude to Dr Ruchi Goel, Dr Pavitra Ganguly, Dr Neelima Gupta, and Dr Smriti Nagpal, for their contributions in the book.

Amit Goel

Contents

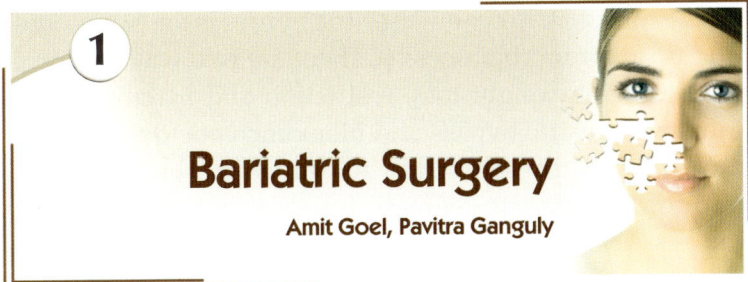

Bariatric Surgery

Amit Goel, Pavitra Ganguly

Bariatric surgery for morbid obesity aims at reducing weight by operative methods.[1] Obesity is defined by body weight that exceeds body weight by 20% and body mass index (BMI) of 30–35 kg/m². Patients with BMI of 35 kg/m² with comorbidities and greater than 40 kg/m² require bariatric surgery. Body mass index measures obesity and is defined by weight/height². Severe obesity is when patient is heavy and fat tissue load creates medical conditions. Currently bariatric surgery is the only long-term effective treatment for obtaining significant weight loss. Laparoscopic Roux-en-Y gastric bypass was first described by Witgroove and colleagues in 1994. Among the different available techniques, the laparoscopic Roux-en-Y gastric bypass is considered gold standard.[2]

Obesity has become a health concern in urban society and is associated with comorbid conditions like hypertension, type 2 diabetes, hyperlipidemia. Severe obesity is defined as BMI greater than 40 or 35 with comorbities like diabetes, hyperlipidemia, and hypertension. Non-surgical treatment of morbid obesity results in regained weight. Surgical therapy as the most successful long-term treatment for morbid obesity. The principle of restricting the volume of oral intake is the basis of gastric stapling procedure. Bariatric surgery for morbid obesity aims at reducing weight by operative means. Roux-en-Y gastric bypass is the commonest procedure for morbid obesity. There are two ways of surgically inducing weight loss, restriction and malabsorption. Roux-en-Y gastric bypass and biliopancreatic diversion are two operative procedures for morbid obesity which incorporate different degrees of malabsorption. Short limb Roux-en-Y is mainly restrictive where as biliopancreatic is restrictive and malabsorptive. The goal of bariatric surgery is improving the health of obese by achieving long-term durable weight loss. It reduces calorie intake, reduced absorption of calories from food and promotes slow ingestion of small boluses of food.

World Health Organisation has defined weight loss surgery of class 1 of BMI of 30–34.9, class 2 of BMI 35–39.9 and class 3 of BMI of 40 and greater than 40. According to American society of metabolic and bariatric surgery the number of Americans undergoing weight loss surgery has increased from 16000 in 1990 to 103000. There is 2.5 fold increase in bariatric procedures from 12800 in 2005 to 31,000 in 2011. Sleeve gastrectomy and gastric bypass are commonest bariatric surgery in France.[3]

Roux-en-Y gastric bypass has proved to be most effective in producing weight loss in severely obese patients. Weight loss after Roux-en-Y gastric bypass ranged from 48 to 74% of excess weight after 5 years of follow-up and more than 50% after 9 years. Roux-en-Y gastric bypass is procedure of choice for patients with a preoperative history suggesting high sugar or sweets intake. It has been the most effective procedure for superobese (greater than 200 pounds over ideal body weight). Roux-en-Y gastric bypass advantage over gastric restrictive operation is that it causes greater sustained weight loss and less difficulty in eating solid food. The disadvantage is absorption of iron, calcium and vitamin B_{12}. Majority weight loss occurred 1 year following surgery and substantial weight loss 3 years after bariatric surgery.

Preoperative medical evaluation requires opinion of physician, dietician and psychologist. Details about weight gain, dietary habits, social situation, and evidence of comorbid diseases. Medical conditions that are caused by obesity are obstructive sleep apnoea, obesity hypoventilation syndrome, asthma, coronary artery disease, atherosclerosis, hypertension, gallbladder disease, GERD, hernias, diabetes, and hyperlipidemia. Screening laboratory tests include complete blood count, electrolytes, liver function tests, iron, vitamin B_{12}, cortisol, thyroid panel, arterial blood gases, bleeding time, clotting time, platelet count, ferritin, albumin, renal function test, calcium, chloride, urinalysis, electrocardiogram and chest X-ray. Ultrasound of abdomen and upper endoscopy are routinely done. Patients with cardiorespiratory conditions must be evaluated. Preoperative and intraoperative criteria prospectively evaluated patient demographics, clinical characteristics, previous abdominal surgery, obesity related comorbidities, hypertension, diabetes, sleep apnoea, coronary disease, stroke, metabolic syndrome and assessment of surgery risk score.[4] Contraindication is hypoventilation syndrome of obesity. The obesity hypoventilation syndrome characterized by hypoxemia, hypercarbia, hypertension and polycythemia. Patients of sleep apnoea, obesity hypoventilation syndrome, asthma should be evaluated by pulmonologist. Patients with gastroesophageal reflux should undergo upper endoscopy for esophagitis and Barrett's esophagus. Nutritional evaluation should be done by dietician. Patients require endocrine, gastroenterology, nephrology and gynaecological consultation. For sweet eaters Roux-en-Y gastric bypass produces greater weight loss due to effects of dumping created by gastrojejunostomy. Rapid weight loss is associated with 30% incidence of gallstone formation. Venous access, intubation, medication doses, anaesthetic doses, arterial gases have to be evaluated. Laparoscopic instrumentations are designed for needs of bariatric patients by extra long trocars and endoscopic staplers. Liver volume was evaluated during the procedure using predefined classification:

1. Small liver volume not impeding exposure.
2. Difficulty in retraction of liver not hindering the passage of instruments or the anastomosis.
3. Difficulty in retraction of liver hindering the passage of instruments but not the anastomosis.
4. Difficulty in retraction of liver, hindering the passage of instruments and gastrojejunal anastomosis.

Operative time was recorded from time of incision and closure of skin. Surgical complications were defined as complication directly related to surgical techniques. Postoperative complications are classified in accordance with Clavien Dindo classification system.[5] Complication occurring between 30 and 90 postoperative days were defined as any complication requiring pharmacological treatment, endoscopic and radiological interventions.

Laparoscopic Roux-en-Y gastric bypass combines restriction and absorption to cause weight loss. Roux-en-Y has minimal malabsorption component compared to other distal bypass. Distal bypass possess increased risk of mineral deficiency and protein calorie malabsorption. The biliopancreatic bypass are examples of 50–150 cm common channels. Using 150 cm Roux-en-Y limb instead of 75–100 cm Roux limb in superobese has found to have greater weight loss. Altering limb length to increase weight loss does not appear to have any long-term benefit except for patients having BMI of 50 and greater than 50.

Another procedure which is done is sleeve gastrectomy which reduces the size of stomach by stapling but preserves the functional stomach which helps for protein digestion and stomach role for satiety. In laparoscopic sleeve gastrectomy

2/3 of stomach is resected and excising greater curvature of stomach leaves a thin tube of stomach that provides restriction. Incidence of diarrhoea, protein malnutrition, bloating, vomiting decrease (Figs 1.1 to 1.9).

Photographs of laproscopic sleeve gastrectomy using staplers:

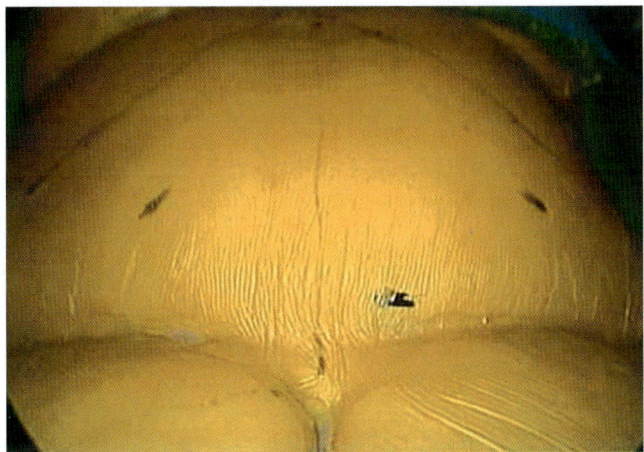

Fig. 1.1

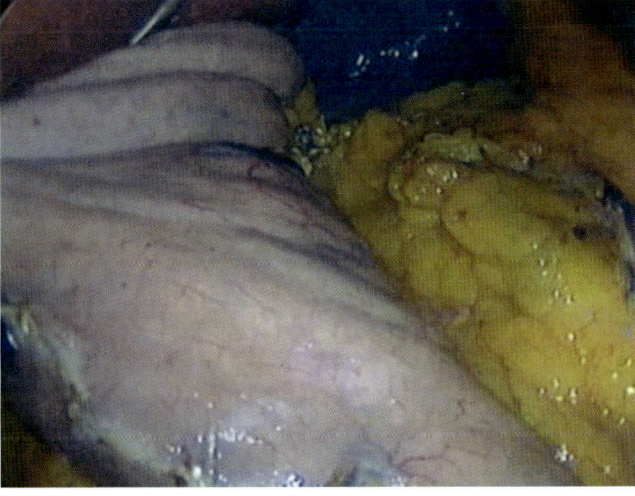

Fig. 1.2

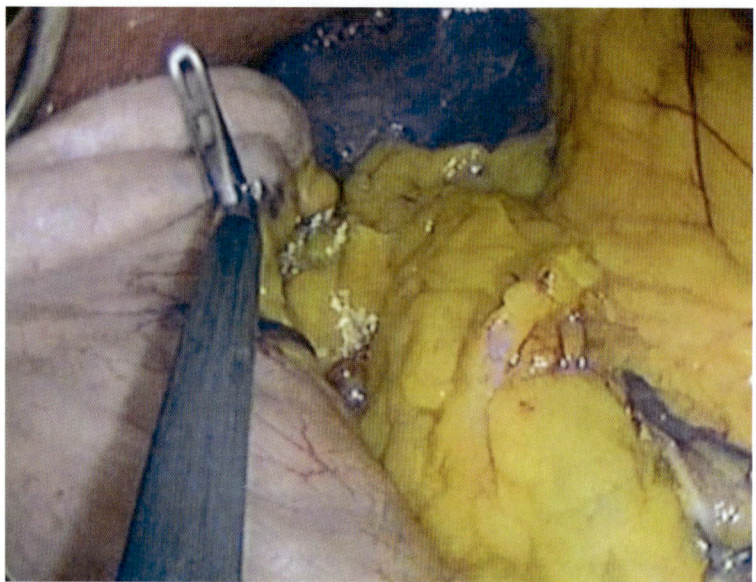

Fig. 1.3

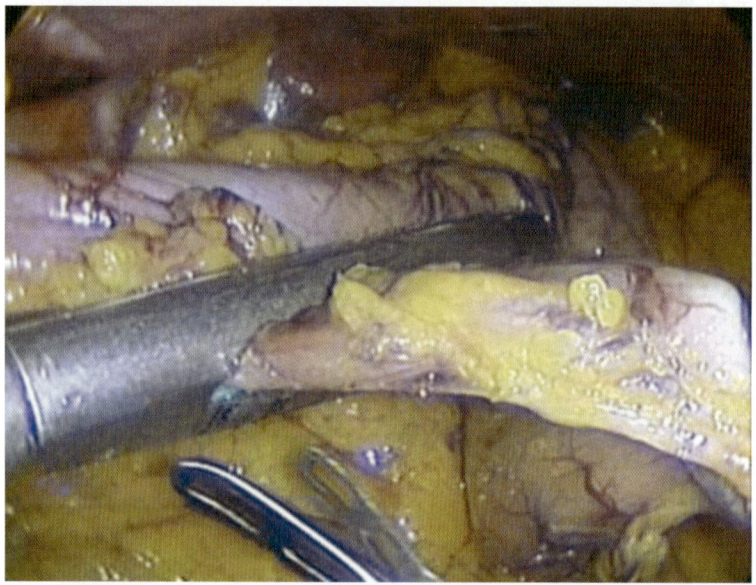

Fig. 1.4

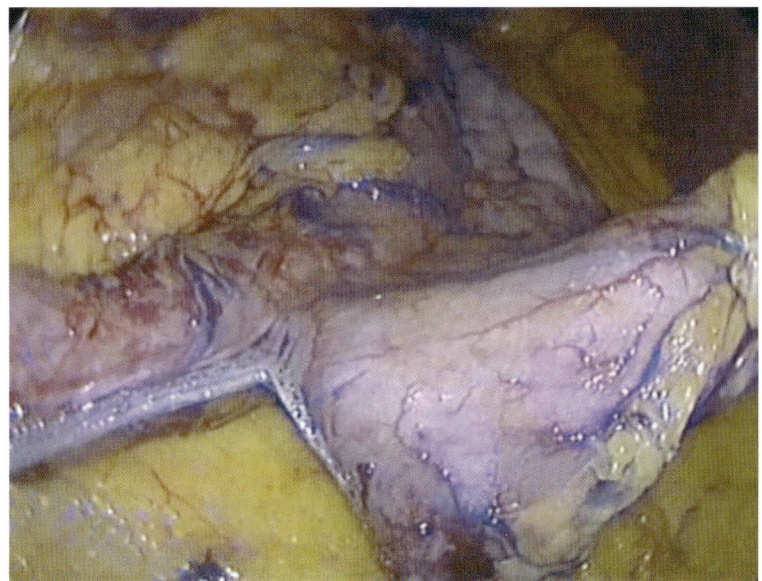

Fig. 1.5

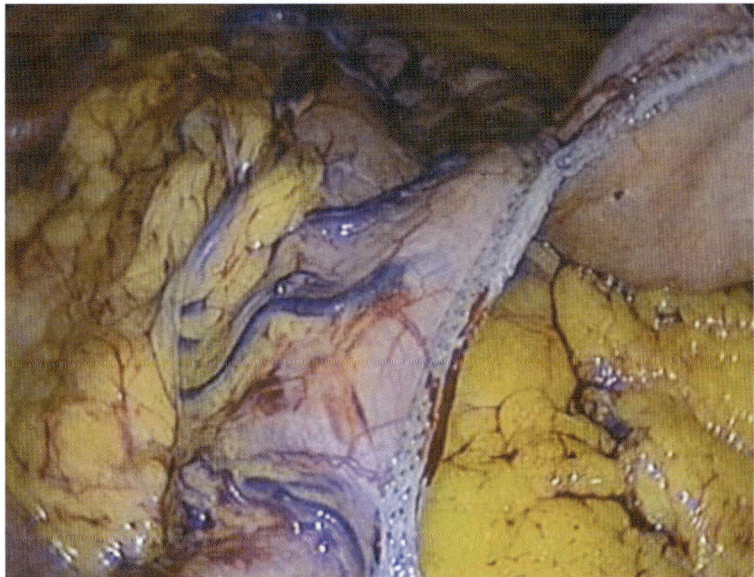

Fig. 1.6

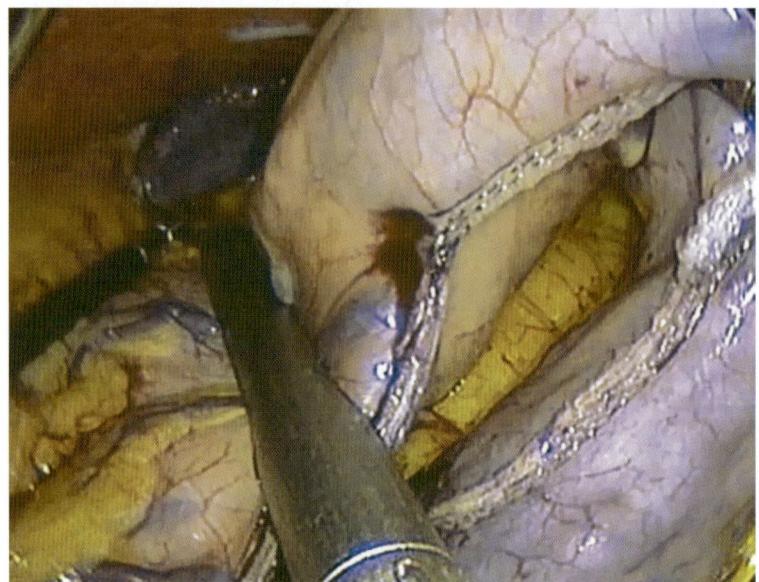

Fig. 1.7

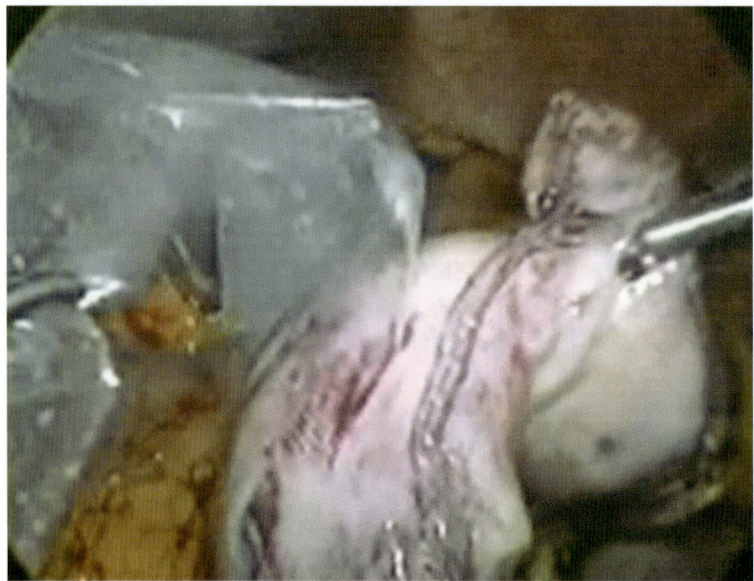

Fig. 1.8

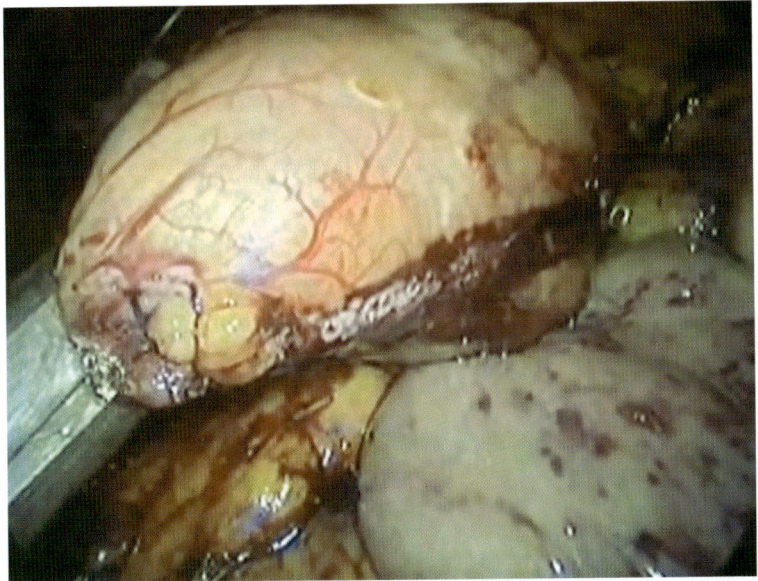

Fig. 1.9

Longer Roux limb is technically difficult to create jejunostomy is smaller calibre. Roux limb longer than 100 cm are used for patients with BMI 50 and above. Anticolic placement of Roux limb appears safe as retrocolic position with lower risk of internal hernia formation.

Retrocolic placement facilitates safe percutaneous access. BPD significantly shortens absorptive surface of intestine, selectively decreases absorption of high calorie fat and alters excessive hormonal response of gut to food intake. Roux-en-Y is less complex and lower incidence of malnutrition yields good results for patients less than 50 kg/m². Preservation of functional stomach by employing sleeve gastrectomy rather than distal partial gastrectomy helps with protein digestion and maintains stomach role in satiety, incidence of diarrhoea, protein malnutrition and bloating.

Malabsorptive procedures include biliopancreatic diversion and biliopancreatic diversion with duodenal switch. BPD is effective for weight loss for individuals with higher body mass index. BPD is efficient for weight loss for individuals with higher body mass index. BPD is efficient procedure to assure maintenance of glycaemic and lipidic metabolic improvement. Biliopancreatic bypass was described by Scopinaro and used for higher BMI patients. Biliopancreatic bypass uses 150 cm Roux limb instead of 75–100 cm Roux limb for gastric bypass. Distal bypass possess increased risk of mineral deficiency and protein calorie malabsorption. BPD is efficient procedure to assure maintenance of glycaemic and lipidic metabolic improvement.

Laparoscopic approach combined with intracorporeal suturing reduces the pulmonary complications, wound complications, lipid complications, decreased hospital stay and postoperative pain. Laparoscopic gastric bypass is technically challenging using laparoscopic procedure. There is video monitor, insufflators, laparoscopic retractors, endoscopic linear staplers, circular staplers, energy sources and endoscopic suturing techniques.

The bariatric tables are designed for accommodating patients greater than 200 lbs weight. Sequential pneumatic compression and deep vein thrombosis prophylaxis are given preoperatively. Sequential compression devices are placed around calves and thighs. Preoperative antibiotics and short acting thrombolytics are administered. Short acting thrombolytics. Bladder catheterization should be done.

Laparoscopes have length of 32–45 cm, angles 0–90 degrees, diameter 5–10 mm, long laparoscope 45 cm. Light source is xenon and metal halide. Insufflators have flow of 30 litres/min. Trocars required are 5, 11, 12, 18 mm.

Laparoscopic instruments are graspers, babcock graspers, bowel clamps and scissors, endoscopic linear staplers, circular staplers. Energy sources are harmonic scalpel and ligature which coagulates 4–6 mm vessels.

PROCEDURE

Surgeon stands between the patient legs with assistant and camera operator on sides. Pneumoperitoneum is established and trocars are placed.

Port arrangement for laparoscopic gastric bypass:

- 5 mm trocar left costal margin
- 5 mm trocar below right costal margin
- 10 mm port left of midline 18 cm below xiphoid
- 5 mm placed left midabdomen
- 12 mm port right midabdomen
- 5 mm subxiphoid left of falciparum

Alternative port arrangement:
- –10 mm, port 15 cm below xiphoid right of midline
- –12 mm, 2–4 cm below and lateral to left rectus
- –5 mm subxiphoid left of falciparum
- –5 mm left costal margin lateral to rectus
- –12 mm right costal margin
- –5 mm left lower quadrant

After placing ports, liver retractor is put and gastrohepatic ligament is opened. Dissection is started 5 cm below gastro-oesophageal junction. Space adjacent to lesser curvature of stomach is cleared to allow passage of endoscopic linear cutting stapler for gastric division. Linear stapler are applied to divide the stomach creating 30 ml proximal gastric pouch that allows creation of gastrojejunostomy. Multiple applications of linear stapler are required from lesser curvature to angle of, has to create proximal pouch of 10–15 cc. Jejunum 75–100 cm distal to ligament of Treitz is divided with endoscopic linear cutting stapler. Mesentery is divided with endoscopic ligatures and endoscopic linear cutting vascular stapler and harmonic scalpel. Stapled side to side enterostomy is made 150 cm distal to this site a 150 cm Roux limb created with side to side jejunostomy with linear endoscopic staplers. For superobese patients an elongated Roux limb of 150–250 cm has been shown for achieving greater weight loss. Window is made in transverse mesocolon to left of middle colic artery and free stapled jejunum of Roux loop is brought to gastric pouch in retrogastric, retrocolic position. Retrocolic route, passing the limb behind mesentery and colon is preferred which takes a direct route. Mesenteric defect is closed to prevent internal herniation. There are numerous ways to perform the gastrojejunostomy, a circular stapled EEA type anastomosis, a stapled side to side anastomosis and hand sewn anastomosis. After completion of gastrojejunostomy, the gastroscope is passed from stomach into small bowel. For circular stapled anastomosis with transoral passage of anvil, upper endoscopy is performed. A percutaneous intravenous cannula is used to introduce loop of wire into lumen of gastric pouch. The endoscope grasps this and attaches it to the anvil of a 21 or 25 mm circular stapler. The anvil is then passed through the oropharynx and esophagus and into the gastric pouch. Electrocautery is applied to stem of the anvil to bring it through the stomach. A left side port is enlarged to allow a circular stapler to be passed. An incision is made through the Roux limb 8 to 10 cm from stapled end to admit the circular stapler which is attached with anvil to create the stapled anastomosis. The enterotomy is closed with linear stapler. Gastrojejunostomy is created by connecting the anvil and shaft of circular stapler and firing the stapler. After anastomotic integrity is established by insufflations of air under saline or by instillation of methylene blue, transverse mesocolic window and fascial defects greater than 5 mm are closed.

Biliopancreatic bypass consists of significant antrectomy with 300 ml gastric pouch. The duodenum is transected. Continuity is restored with long alimentary limb and relatively short common channel through which bile and pancreatic secretions are drained with intestinal contents.

Duodenal switch procedure consists of sleeve resection of stomach with preservation of pylorus. For biliopancreatic diversion the surgeon operates from patients left side to perform the common channel and between legs to do antrectomy and gastrojejunostomy. Ileocaecal junction is identified and 50 cm proximal to it is marked with silk suture. From this point, another 150 cm proximally is identified and transacted the intestine with endoscopic linear stapler. Patient is placed in reverse Trendlenburg position, devascularize the greater curve by harmonic scalpel. Create window in gastrohepatic ligament and divide the pylorus with 60 × 35 mm stapler for endoscopic gastrointestinal anastomosis. Devascularise the lesser curve of stomach and divide the stomach using firing of 60 × 3.5 mm stapler. Divide the omentum with harmonic till the transverse colon. Using harmonic scalpel create a gastrotomy posterior to staple line on stomach. Place the alimentary limb to greater curve of stomach to facilitate stapling of gastrojejunostomy. Enterotomy is closed and anastomosis is tested with methylene blue.

Complications

Complications of laparoscopic gastric bypass are intestinal leak due to anastomotic leak, staple line disruption, perforation, pulmonary embolus, acute gastric dilatation, internal herniation, marginal ulcer, stomal stenosis, internal hernia. After gastric bypass sugars cause dumping syndrome. Symptoms include bloating, cramps, sweating, hypotension.

Diet

Preoperatively patient is advised to drink clear liquids day before surgery. After gastric bypass patient is discharged and told to drink fluids, focus on eating proteins, take short walks 6–8 times a day. Pain management, activity alleviates discomfort. Sodas, candy, aerated drinks, sweetened cereals, caffeine should not be taken after bariatric surgery. Nutritional requirement includes protein 75 g/day, carbohydrates 100 g/day, fats 50 g/day, water 2 litre/day, vitamins, calcium and iron. Initially clear sugar free liquids are started and from 2 to 8 months pureed semisolid food is allowed. A diet of 600–800 calories with 75 g protein should be taken for initial months. Patient is advised to eat at mealtimes. Fluids should be drunk before meals and hour after meals. Three small protein meals should be taken. Patient is advised to eat small meals and do not snack between meals. Liquids ½ cup every hour and multivitamins, calcium, iron should be taken regularly. Foods difficult to chew bread products, cow milk products, pasta products, fatty foods, fried foods, candy, chocolate, carbonated beverages, bran cereals, corn, beans, coconut should not be taken.

Patients lose 65–80% excess weight within 12–18 months after bariatric surgery. People with clinically severe obesity, bariatric surgery is the best option. Gastric bypass surgery is time tested endorsed by consensus panel conveyed by national institute of health. Vitamin, minerals and high protein intake are required for nutritional deficiencies. Duodenal switch, biliopancreatic diversion is method for achieving weight loss for extremely obese with BMI—50 kg/m^2 but

brings higher rates of malnutrition. Restrictive gastric procedures restrict the size of stomach. Silastic ring gastroplasties
restrict the size of stomach. Overweight people between
BMI—25–30 would benefit from exercising 45 minutes 3 times
a week would lose 18% excess weight.

Recent Literature

Meta-analysis of 6587 patients to evaluate 12–24 months
impact of bariatric surgery on type 2 diabetes, hypertension
and hyperlipidemia, there is BMI reduction of 5 after surgery,
type 2 diabetes reduction of 33%, hypertension reduction of
27%. Bariatric surgery is effective therapeutic option to
reduce cardiovascular risk in severely obese patients.[6]

Jacobson HJ studied 2000 patients who underwent
laparoscopic gastric bypass. Mean time was 102 minutes,
complication rates 2.8% and hospital stay was 3 days.[7]

Padwal Klasenbach did medline search of 2619 patients
managed by bariatric surgery. The difference for BMI was
11.4% for jejunoileal bypass, 10.1 for sleeve gastrectomy, 9.0
for Roux-en-Y gastric bypass.[8]

Recent meta-analysis shows 62–70% excess weight loss
following gastric bypass, diabetes was resolved in 76.8%.
Bariatric surgery recommended for patient with BMI 40 and
medical conditions sleep apnoea, cardiomyopathy and
diabetes improves.[9]

Reoch conducted randomized trials comparing laparoscopic and open bariatric surgery. Laparoscopic surgery was
associated with lower risk of wound infection 0.21%,
incisional hernia 0.11%, reoperation 1.06% and anastomotic
leaks 0.64%.[10]

American society of metabolic and bariatric surgery efforts
to assess programmatic quality in bariatric centres. It plans
to analyse centres outcomes based on ORS–MRS to collect

data to facilitate bariatric surgery and scoring system for risk evaluation. Class C patients with 4, 5 comorbidities with morbid obesity were considered high risk.[11]

According to the Organization for Economic Cooperation and Development Health Data 2012, obesity rate percentage of total adult population with BMI 30 kg/m² was 26. 1% in UK, 35.9% in USA and only 3.5% in Japan.[12]

Bariatric surgery is the most effective long-term treatment for patients suffering from higher degrees of obesity. Metabolic operations deeply influence hormonal secretion especially in proximal part of small bowel, change parameters of entero-insular axis having influence on insulin secretion and complex of glucose tolerance.[13]

Another technique to perform Roux-en-Y gastric bypass is by robotic surgery. Since 2001 robotic surgery has been introduced to operating room to perform digestive surgical procedures and its use is constantly rising despite high costs.[14]

References

1. Winlock G, Levington S, Sherliker P, et al. Body mass index and cause specific mortalty in 900000 adults collaborative analysis of 57 prospective studies Lancet 2009; 373: 1083–96.

2. Powell MS, Fernandez AZ, et al. Surgical treatment for morbid obesity, the laparoscopic Roux-en-Y gastric bypass. Surg Clin North Am 2011; 91: 1203–24.

3. Lazzati A, Laucher R, Delarina V, et al. Bariatric surgery trends in France. Surg Obes Relat Dis 2013; Aug 26.

4. Demaria EJ, Portemier D, Woefe L. Obesity surgery mortality risk of proposal for a clinical useful score to predict mortality risk of patients undergoing gastric bypass. Surg Obes Relat Dis 2007; 3: 134–40.

5. Dindo D, Demartine N, Clavien PA. Classification of surgical complication, a new proposal with evaluation in a cohort of 6336 patients and results of a survey. Ann Surg 2004; 240: 205–13.

6. Ricci C, Gaeta M, Rausa C, et al. Early impact of bariatric surgery on type 2 diabetes, hypertension and hyperlipidemia, a systemia review, meta-analysis and meta-regression. Obes Surg 2013, Nov 10.

7. Jacobson HJ, Burgland A, Roeder J, Gislason et al. High Volume bariatric surgery in a single centre, safety, quality, cost efficacy and teaching aspects in 2000 consecutive cases. Obes Surg Relat Dis 2011;Nov 25.

8. Padwal R, Klesenbach S, Wobe N, et al. Safety of laparoscopic vs open bariatric surgery, a systemic review and network meta-analysis of randomized trials. Obes rev 2011 Aug;12(8): 602–21.

9. Zhao Y, Encinosa W. Healthcare cost and utilization project 2006–2007, Jan.

10. Reoch J, Mottilo S, Shinony A, et al. Safety of laproscopic vs open bariatric surgery, a systemic review and meta-analysis. Arch Surg 2011 Nov;146(11): 1314–22.

11. Coloquitt J, Clegg A, Loveman E. Surgery for morbid obesity, Cochrane database syst Rev 2005;(4) CD003641.

12. Organisation for economic cooperation and development OECD health data 2012, OECD, Paris 2012.

13. Fried M, Minerva Endocrinol 2013 Sep;38(3):237–44.

14. Maesco S, Reza M, Mayol JA. Efficiency of the da vinci surgical system in abdominal surgery compared with laparoscopy, a systemic review and meta-analysis. Ann Surg 2010; 252:254–62.

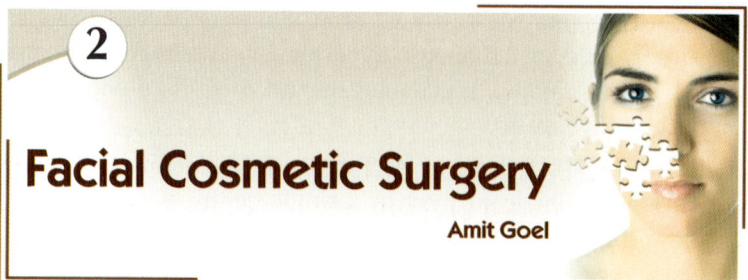

2

Facial Cosmetic Surgery

Amit Goel

Modern era of aesthetic surgery began about 1900.[1, 2] Rhinoplasty reported by Dieffenbach in 1845 and breast augmentation with lipoma graft by Czerny in 1895.[3, 4] The first endonasal rhinoplasty, blepharoplasty and surgery to eliminate wrinkles was published by surgeons from developing world.[5] Three German surgeons: Hollander (1901), Lexer (1906), and Joseph (1912) claimed first facial cosmetic case.[6, 7] Facial fat grafting was reported by German physician Franz Neuber in 1893.[8] Madam Noel was famous aesthetic surgeon of her times. She performed face lifts and blepharoplasties. Surgical treatment of forehead and temporal area has been described by Hunt and Madam Noel pioneers of facial aesthetic surgery in 1926.[9, 10]

FACE

Face is divided into
- Upper face
- Midface
- Lower face and neck

Upper third of face lies above the lateral canthal angle and includes forehead, eyebrows and upper eyelids. The middle third of face lies between lateral canthal angle and nasolabial fold. This includes lateral canthal tendon, medial canthal tendon, skin, fat, orbicularis oculi muscle, suborbicularis oculi fat pad, malar fat pad, orbitomalar ligament, orbital septum, zygomaticus major, minor muscles and levator labii superioris. The lower third of face includes structures below nasolabial fold. Upper face is forehead and temporal region. Mid-face extends from corner of mouth to corner of eye, skin, fat, muscle of cheek. Lower face is below corner of mouth. Patients prioritize their aging concentration along the lines of these surgical units which helps the surgeon deciding about sequencing for surgery. Subcutaneous fat in the face and neck is separated into superficial and deep layers by fascia superficialis, SMAS. Fascia superficialis is called temporoparietal fascia and galea in the temporal region and forehead and SMAS in midface and neck. Superficial fat is tightest in forehead, temporal and loosening on descending on face, cheek and neck regions. Fat superficial to SMAS comprises 56% of total fat in humans. Superficial fat is densest around nasolabial folds. Fat deep to SMAS less abundant and comprises 44% of total facial fat. Deep fat is densest in temporal, periocular region. Eighty percent of fat is in face and 20% in neck. Superficial fat is continuous and densest in cheek. The true retaining ligaments anchor dermis to periosteum sags are located over zygomaticofrontal suture, zygomatic arch body suture. False retaining ligaments anchor superficial fascia to deep fascia are located in anterior, middle and posterior cheek. Fascial architecture is concentric arrangement of layers consisting of skin, superficial fascia, superficial SMAS, mimetic musculature with deep fat. SMAS is fibromuscular network lying deep to dermis and superficial to fascial moter nerves extending from superficial temporal musculature to platsyma below. SMAS is functional muscular activity and lifting subcutaneous tissues of face and neck. The main trunk and branches of fascial nerve are below zygomatic arch. The fascial muscles are layered into superficial and deep fascia and work synchronously. Sensory supply of face and neck is primarily through branches of trigeminal and cervical plexus.

AGING

Fascial aging is result of progressive gravimetric tissue descent and causes are solar elastosis. Dermis begins to lose collagen and elastin. Fat increases occurs in face in regions called depots deep to superficial fascia. These depots are in abdomen, hips, thighs and flanks. Face and neck have highest concentration of glandular and lymphatic tissue which accounts for firmness. Glandular tissues of face shrink with aging. Laxity of orbital retaining ligaments and septa cause crows feet, lower eyelid bags and festoons. Sphincter action of orbicularis muscle causes crows feet. Skeleton resorption of anterior fascial skeleton especially in pyriform and inferior orbital rim region contributing to appearance of aged face. Fine superficial lines in skin are called wrinkles. Deep wrinkles are called mimetic lines. They require multimodality therapy. Skin folds require surgical tightening procedure called blepharoplasty, brow lift and face lift. Frontalis muscle tightening and thickening cause worry lines or horizontal forehead lines. Procerus or corrugators muscle hypertrophy causes frown lines. Midfacial descent behind mandibular retaining ligaments creates jowls. Upper eyelid skin sages, loses elasticity. There is lateral hooding because of descent of eyebrows. Horizontal lines or wrinkles become continuous, nasal tip descends and tissue accumulates around neck. There are changes in thickness of fascial skin, skin of cheek, nasal lobule. Forehead lines become thicker, lower eyelid and nose become thinner. 1% of collagen diminishes per year of adult life.[11] Collagen diminishes and there is significant increase of skin thickness and abundance of thickened degraded elastic fibres. Melanocytes diminish and there is decrease of normal depth of dermal epidermal papillae.

There are fewer sebaceous glands, pigment and hair shafts. There is deleterious effect of sunlight on skin. Sequela of ultraviolet radiation causes thicker skin, increased ground substance, proliferation of elastic fibres, mechanical bending and stretching of skin along lines of force determined by insertions and attachments of underlying fascial muscles.

Surgical Rejuvenation

Surgeon uses guidelines for patient assessment and analysing patients features, advising about surgical correction.

Primary indication of surgical rejuvenation of upper face is soft tissue ptosis of forehead, brow and temporal regions. Coronal brow lift is for deep glabellar and forehead lines. Face lift is incision around the ear extending partially around neck, jaws, mouth and nasolabial folds. Bianchi has stated that facelift is widely used for rhytidectomy, parotidectomy and mandibular resections.[12] Temporal lift is offered for older patients with lateral brow ptosis and extensive crows feet. Endoscopic brow lift is for middle aged patient with glabellar frown lines and brow ptosis. Coronal brow lift is for deep glabellar and forehead lines. For temporal lifts initial dissection within the hairline is performed in subgaleal plane followed by subperiosteal plane. Optimal temporal flap mobilization, subperiosteal dissection of lateral orbit and zygoma is necessary. Coronal lifts is performed with pretrichal and scalp incision. Extensive and continuous excision of fat in submental and submandibular areas through submental and rhytidectomy incisions forms basis of face lifts.

Browpexy are superciliary incisions given to elevate brow. Brow repositioning consists of excising skin and tissue from midforehead. Procedure is excision of forehead skin and subcutaneous tissue between transverse forehead coronal. Vermilion advancement is carried for patients with long upper lip with wedge of skin.

Malar implants have been placed for patients having flat midface. They add bulk to face and are inserted through temporal subperiosteal exposure. Submental and buccal fat could be resected by rhytidectomy. Otoplasty is done for aesthetic ear lobule. Midfacial lift relied on elevating of midface by superotemporal approach by coronal incision. Endoscopic approach is called coronacanthoplasty. Similar midface lifts have been described by extended infraciliary incision. Midface lift has emphasised on lifting suborbicularis oculi fat pad. Subperiosteal midface lift with release of periosteum is needed for powerful midface lift. When full thickness midface advancement is performed with PTFE orbital rim implant midface rejuvenation occurs.

Endoscopic subperiosteal lifting elevates entire cheek mass. Malar fat pad is lifted for superior lateral direction. Current approach for midface rejuvenation combines use of percutaneous suture technique lifting cheek fat pad. Small temporal incision with elevation in anterior and inferior direction. Dissection is carried from lateral canthus and sentinel vein cauterized. Fat transfer to midface is by lipostructure and fat autograft muscle injection. Endoscopic face lift is by temporal fascia. Recently polyethylene implant has been used.

Z Plasty is for relaxing contracted scars. Size of each angle is 60° constructed that two triangles have shape of parallelograms. Single Z plasty achieves 2 cm of lengthening and multiple Z plasty achieves 0.5 cm of length for each Z plasty.

Chemical peels and dermabrasion are cosmetic procedures for facial lines. Dermabrasion is removal of epidermis and dermis and used for removing facial scars. It improves glabellar creases and beneficial for acne and scars. Elderly patients wih light complexion who have extensive wrinkling due to sun exposure benefits from chemical peels. Wrinkles treated by chemical peels and creases treated by dermabrasion. Chemical peels are tricloracetic solution, phenol, green soap, croten. Effective dealing with creases is cutting muscles that cause them.

Botox injections are advised for dynamic forehead and glabellar lines. Material threaded through skin creases are called fillers. Vicryl, catgut, resected SMAS, silicon, fat, collagen were used. When forehead and glabellar lines are static and appear with dermal furrows soft tissue fillers and laser resurfacing should be offered. Botulinum toxin improves facial appearance, protrusion of muscle bulk and alteration of facial units. Several types of facial wrinkling that becomes pronounced with age, gravitational redundancy, volume loss redundancy, loss of skin elasticity, sleep creases and dynamic facial lines. Dynamic lines induced by muscle contraction are amenable to botulinum toxin treatment. Botulinum are neurotoxins produced by gram-positive anaerobic bacterium. Two commercial botulinum toxins (botox, allergen immune CA) and myobloc elan pharmaceuticals San Diego CA. Dyport (Berkshire UK) Botox unit is 3–5 times potent than dysport unit. Each vial of botox contains 100 mu of *Clostridium botulinum*. For cosmetic uses concentration vary from 1 unit per 0.1 ml to 10 U per 0.1 ml. Dysport is suppled by 500 U vials. Botulinum toxin is administered by injection into target muscle, to choose the site of injection to treat wrinkles, patient is asked to squeeze and relax the muscles of affected area. Surgeon identifies location of maximal skin displacement during contraction of muscle. The solution is injected in muscle rather than crease lines. The effects of botox are temporary and resolve between 2 and 11 months. Subsequent injections could have different duration of effect. Dramatic responses are seen for patients between 30 and 50 years where injections will flatten the edges of indentation. Deeper wrinkles, treatment with botulinum will flatten edges but additional filler techniques required to make area smooth. Preinjection councilling for side effects of botox are told. Botox is supplied through bottles of 100 units and injections are given with 1 ml syringe with 30 gauge needle. Smoking and sun exposure accentuate the depth of wrinkles. Doses of botox depends on site of wrinkles (Fig. 2.1).

The glabellar area is commonly treated area. Glabellar folds develop from contractions of corrugators, orbicularis

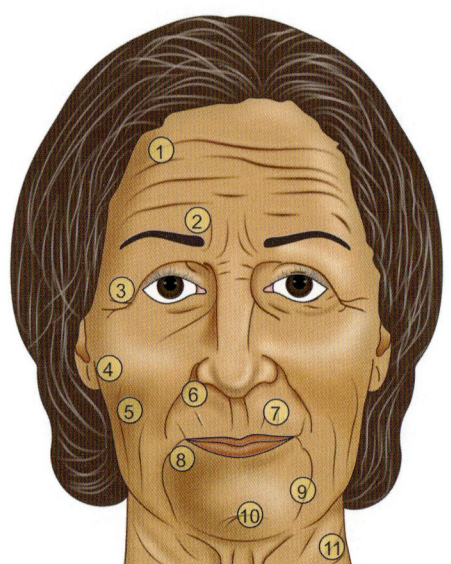

1. Worry lines　　　2. Frown lines　　　3. Crown lines
4. Preauricular lines　5. Cheek lines　　　6. Nasolabial lines
7. Lip lines　　　　8. Commissural lines 9. Marionette lines
10. Chin lines　　　11. Neck lines

Fig. 2.1: Commonly seen facial wrinkles

and procerus muscles. Vertical folds are from the corrugators and the horizontal folds are from procerus. The patient squeezes these muscles and the bulges are marked per injection. Usually 4–5 mm lateral to vertical wrinkles lines. concentration used is 2.5 to 10 U per 0. 1 ml, volume injected is 0.05 to 0.1 ml. The total dose for glabellar region is 20–30 U (Fig. 2.2).

Injections are given 1 cm above the brow area to prevent brow ptosis. The forehead is treated lateral to the centre of brow with lower doses than central forehead. The concentration is 2.5–5 U/ml, volume is 0.025 ml/site, total dose is 10–20 U (Fig. 2.3).

Injection for lateral periocular rhytides/crows feet are fanned along the lateral orbital rim. Doses are 7.515 U per side. Infiltration is 0.3–0.5 ml of 2.5 ml/0.1 ml (Fig. 2.4).

Injection for brow repositioning the sites are extended from orbicularis along the lateral superior orbital rim and under the brow. Superficial injections are 2.5–5 U/0.1 ml. Volume is 0.025–0.05 ml/per site into 3–5 sites/side (Fig. 2.5).

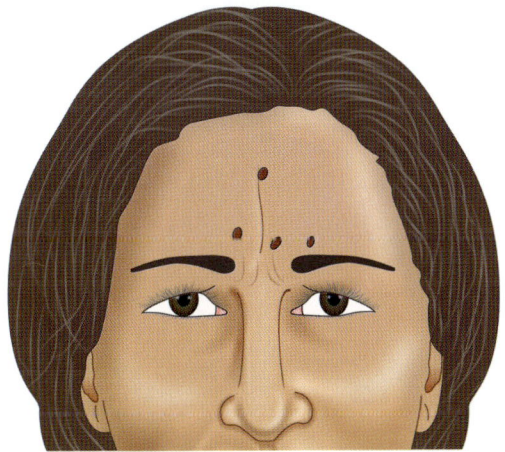

Fig. 2.2: Injection sites for glabellar region

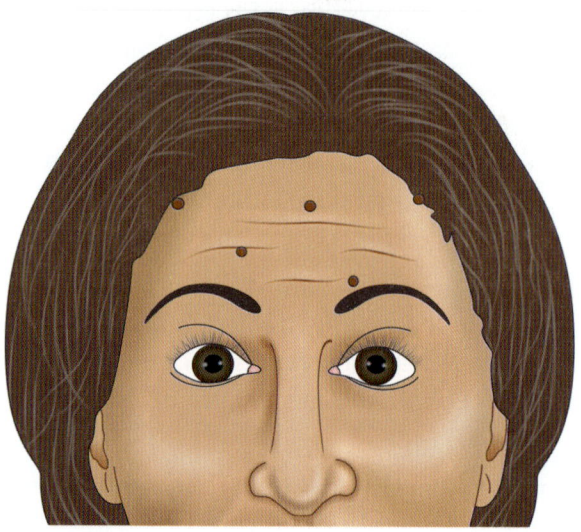

Fig. 2.3: Injection sites for horizontal forehead wrinkles

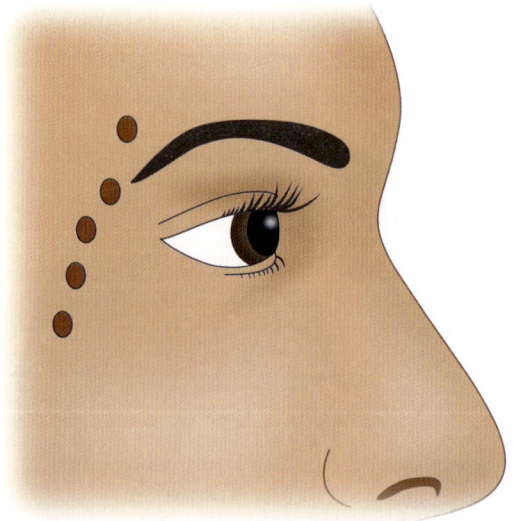

Fig. 2.4: Injection for lateral periocular rhytides/crows feet are fanned along the lateral orbital rim

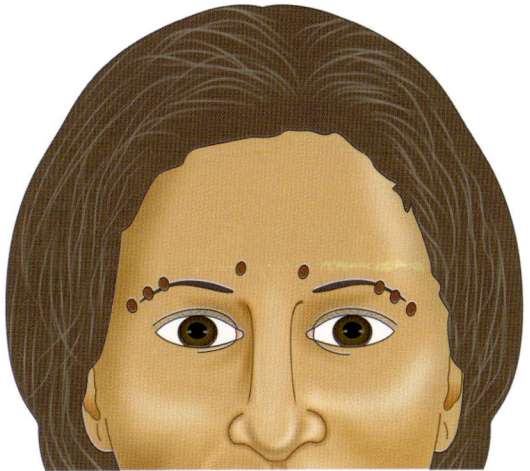

Fig. 2.5: Injection sites for brow repositioning

Injection sites for orbicularis ridge is concentration of 2.5 to 1 U/0.1 ml. The volume injected is 0.025–0.05/per site (Fig. 2.6).

Injection sites for perioral wrinkles lines are placed just above the vermilion. These are produced because of contraction of orbicularis oris. Doses are 2.5 U per 0.1 ml and less than 0.025 to 0.05 ml injected per site (Fig. 2.7).

Melobial folds is technique dependent and are injected 1–2.5 U per 0.1 ml and 0.05 ml injected per site (Fig. 2.8).

Platysmal folds require 2.5–10 U per 0.1 and 0.05–0.1 ml injected per site and 30–100 U are injected (Fig. 2.9).

Fillers is human collagen prepared from human donor tissue processed from cadavers. Injections are painful and 20% overcorrection is required. Dermalogen is the human collagen is infiltrated continuously in beading fashion. Chemodenervation reduces dynamic component and collagen treats static component.

Patients prioritize their aging concern along the lines of surgical units which helps the surgeon deciding about sequencing for surgery.

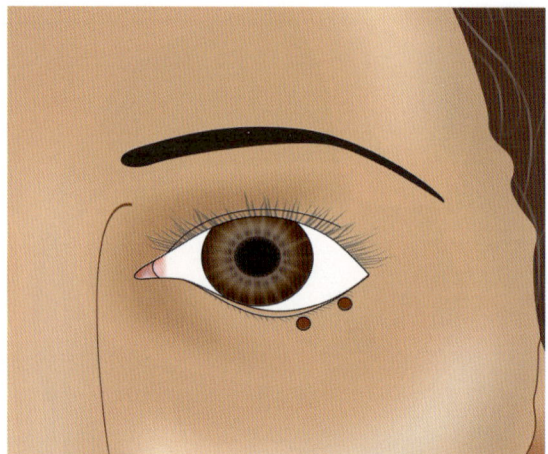

Fig. 2.6: Injection sites for orbicularis ridge

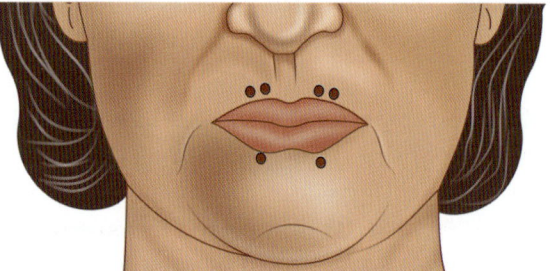

Fig. 2.7: Injection sites for periocular wrinkles lines

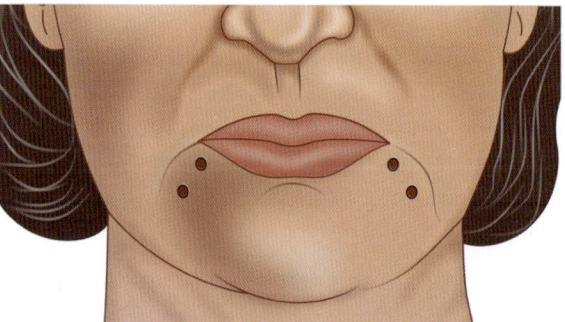

Fig. 2.8: Injection sites for mesolabial lines

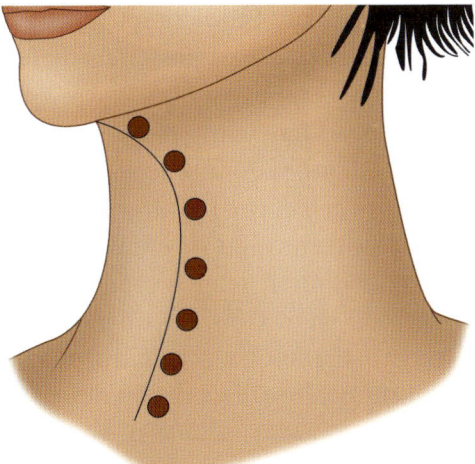

Fig. 2.9: Injection sites for platysmal bands

Recent Literature

Mean reduction of apparent age for cosmetic surgical patients was 6 years. Facelift surgical procedures causes reduction of 4.6 years, laser facelift was 2.5 years, endoscopic forehead lift was 2 years.[13]

Smoking causes facial aging, affects middle, lower thirds of face with 5 years difference between smokers and non-smokers.[14]

47 patients underwent facelift and per oral peel and patients were evaluated on outcome measurement. patients postoperative age was 8.2 younger than real age.[15]

Fat was used for filler material to correct facial volume loss. Fat is ideal subcutaneous filler because it is living and removed if overcorrection occurs. Facial fat grafting done with injection control device.[16]

Tissue expansion is used for repairing large scalp defects.[17]

Skin expansion is major development in reconstructive surgery. The use of tissue expansion is method of choice for congenital and acquired defects. Study analysed 35 expansion procedures for 35 patients. Study helps for drawing attention on different aspects of tissue expansion using tissue expanded and smooth surface tissue expanders.[18]

Expanded forehead flap using temporal pedicles are used extensively for facial reconstruction. Distal expanded forehead flaps are used for hemifacial reconstruction to overcome the disadvantage of dual temporal pedicles, limited transfers and short length of flaps.[19]

Adipose derived stem cells, pleuripotent cells found in stroma of adipose tissues contribute to recovery by promoting wound healing. Facial skin defect repair without skin grafts provide rapid coverage of wound with patients own regenerated skin.[20]

Vascularized composite allotransplantation multiple types of tissues are transferred from donor to recipient performed for upper extremity, face and abdomen. 70 patients underwent upper extremity and face transplants. Vascularized composite allotransplantation is emerging field which provides avenues for reconstructive procedures.[21]

5199 patients underwent infiltration of cryopreserved fat for nasolabial folds and lips. Outcomes were satisfactory and improved contour.[22]

References

1. Rogers BO. A brief history of cosmetic surgery. Surg Clin North America 1971;51:256.

2. Stephenson KL. The history of blepharoplasty to correct blepharochalasi. Aesthetic Plast Surg 1971;1:17.

3. Czerny VU. Plasticher ersatz der brustdrüse durch em lipom zentralbl chir 1895;27:72.

4. Roe JO. The deformity termed pig nose and its correlation by subcutaneous operation. Plast Reconstr Surg 1900;42:78.

5. Miller CC. The excision of bag-like folds of skin from the region about the eyes. Med Brief 1906;34:648.

6. Hollander E. Plastische kosmetische operation kristsche klemperen neuve deutsche climex vol9 urban and schwartigen Berlin 1932.

7. Joseph J. Hangewangenplastik meleomiplastice dtch med wechenschr 1921;47:287.

8. Neuber F, Fettransplantation NF, Chir Kongr Verhandl. Dtsch Ges Chir 1893;22–66.

9. Hunt L. Plastic surgery of head, face and neck. Lea and Febinger, Philadelphia 1926.

10. Noel. La churugie, Esthetique et sa role sociale maso et cie Paris 1926.

11. Frenske NA, Lober CW. Structural and functional changes of normal aging skin. Jam acad dermatol 1986;15:571.

12. Bianchi B, Ferri A, Copelli C, et al. Head and neck 2013; Aug 30.

13. Swanson E, Objective assessment of change of apparent age after facial rejuvenation surgery, J Plast Reconstr Aesthet 2011 Sept; 64(9):1124–31.

14. Okada HC, Alleyne B, Varghai K, et al. Facial changes caused by smoking, a comparison between smoking and non-smoking identical twins. Plast Reconstr Surg 2013; Aug 6.

15. Ozturk CN, Huettner F, Ozturk C, et al. Objective assessment of combination facelift and perioral phenol croton oil peel. Plast Reconst Surg 2013 Nov;132(5):143.

16. Hugh E, Hetherington Jon E, Boce K. Complications from laser assisted Clin Cosmet investing dermatol 2013;6(6):201–9.

17. Gan C, Fan J, Liu L. Reconsconstruction of large unilateral hemifacial scar contractures with supercharged expanded forehead flaps based on anterofrontal superficial temporal vessels. J Plast Reconst Aesthet Surg 2013; Jul 27.

18. Manquibat EA. Facial Plast Surg Clin North Am 2013 Aug 21; (3):487 96.

19. Yesilada AK, Akeal A, Dagdelin D, et al. The feasibility of tissue expansion in reconstruction of congenital and acquired

deformities of paediatric patients. Int J Burns Trauma 2013 July 8;3(3):144–50.

20. Jo Di, Yang HJ, Kim SH, et al. Coverage of skin defects without skin grafts using adipose derived stem cells. Aesthet Plast Surg 2013 July 23.

21. Murphy BD, Zuker RM, Borschel GH. Vascularized composite allotransplantation, an update on medical and surgical progress and remaining challenges. J Plast Reconst Aethet Surg 2013 July 15.

22. Erol OO, Agyoglu G. Aesthetic Surg J 2013 Jul;33(5):639–53.

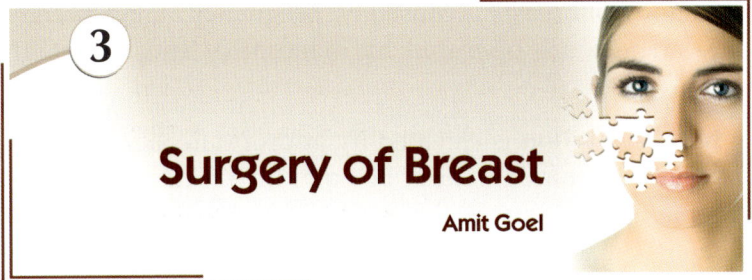

Surgery of Breast

Amit Goel

Surgery of breast involves changing shape and size of breast. Cosmetic surgery of breast involves reduction mammoplasty and mastopexy. Operations are primarily at decreasing the size of breasts (reduction mammoplasty) and reconstruction. Extremely large breast create physical and psychological problems. Physical problems include neck and back pain, posture related problems, grooves of shoulders, numbness of arms and skin problems within inframammary folds. The goal of reduction mammoplasty is to reduce the size of breasts, elevate the nipple and preserve the blood supply to nipple areola complex.

Nipple areola complex is attached to pedicle of underlying breast tissue. These procedures are described by orientation of pedicle.

Small breasts could be enlarged by breast augmentation called augmentation mammoplasty. Breast implants are placed directly beneath breast tissue (subglandular) beneath pectoralis major. Implants are constructed of outer silicon shell filled with saline. The common problem of implant is breast firmness which results from excessive scar tissue and from capsule that forms around implants. Capsular contracture cause symptoms for 15% patients.

Sagging of breasts is caused by pregnancy, aging, weight loss surgery are operated by mastopexy and breast lift operations.

Nipple position is elevated by appropriate skin incision. Breast augmentation could be combined with mastopexy. Augmentation is surgical procedure used to increase size of womans breasts using breast implants. Woman could choose to enhance their figure by breast augmentation. Breast surgery enlargement begins with incision at crease of breasts. A space is created underneath breast tissue under chest muscle. Saline and silicon implants are usually placed of which silicon implants are commoner. Breast tissue covered by insurers. It carries risk of 1–3% infection, 1–3% haematoma and scarring. Implants are placed between beneath the pectoralis major of chest. Saline is injected progressively to expand the tissues. Silicon implants are commonly placed in 70% cases. Breast reconstruction is covered by insurers in many countries.

RECONSTRUCTIVE BREAST SURGERY

Reconstruction after mastectomy is routinely done. Breast augmentation is achieved by silicon implant. The commonest approach is incision in inframammary fold of breast. The implant is placed deep to pectoral muscles. Complications include haematomas, infection, capsular contracture, leakage of silicon into tissues. Breast reduction is where breast tissue and skin is excised and then reconstructed by mobilizing breast tissue from either side. Symmetry of breast size and shape are important and nipple and areola are positioned. Complications include nipple necrosis.

Simultaneous breast reconstruction: Women have immediate reconstruction when they are having their mastectomy.

Staged breast reconstruction: Women who require radiation are advised staged breast reconstruction.

Delayed breast reconstruction: Women who require cosmetic breast reconstruction which is inserting silicon or saline implants underneath chest muscle. Breast reconstruction with flap procedures are done by reconstructive surgeons where breast is reconstructed using tissue taken from abdomen, back, buttocks, thighs which are transplanted to chest by reconnecting blood vessels of chest by micro-surgery.

Breast reconstruction could be accomplished by technique called flap reconstruction. Flap reconstruction are placed at back, buttocks, thigh, abdomen. The latissimus dorsi muscle flaps are common flaps for reconstruction of breasts. Abdominal flaps for breast reconstruction are TRAM flaps (transverse rectus abdominis myocutaneous flaps). Muscle sparing latissimus dorsi flap is reliable and efficient technique for autologous breast reconstruction.[1] Augmentation mammoplasty are common surgical procedures. Breast implants have texture and give aesthetic results.[2]

Breast reconstruction is common cosmetic surgical procedure where implants are placed under chest muscle which provides better support. Subglandular implants are placed under breast gland and incision are either axillary or transumbilical. Complications are infection, haematoma, capsule formation. Silicon is silicon carbon-based polynet used for breast implants. Breast reconstruction follow breast cancer surgery and immediate reconstruction is regarded gold standard. Pedicled flaps are latissimus dorsi based on thoracodorsal vessels. TRAM flaps are commonest reconstruction flaps for breast reconstruction. The flap could be pedicled on superior pedicle, superior epigastric artery and inferior pedicle on inferior epigastric artery.

Free flap breast reconstruction using microvascular techniques. TRAM flaps are based on deep inferior epigastric artery that could be anastomosed to contralateral internal thoracic or ipsilateral thoracodorsal artery (Fig. 3.1). Free flaps require less muscle but produce better breast shape. Older procedures (TRAM flaps and latissimus dorsi flaps) causes higher risk of hernia, abdominal bulging and limiting of physical activity.

Transverse rectus abdominis flap is constructive option in postmastectomy breast reconstruction. The flap is pedicle based on superior pedicle. It could be used for breast reconstruction using microvascular techniques by free flap. Superior epigastric artery is artery supplying the flap. TRAM flap is taken with inferior pedicle using microvascular techniques. Deep inferior epigastric artery forms the vascular basis of flap. Newer flaps used for breast reconstruction are tissue expanders, deep inferior artery perforator flap,

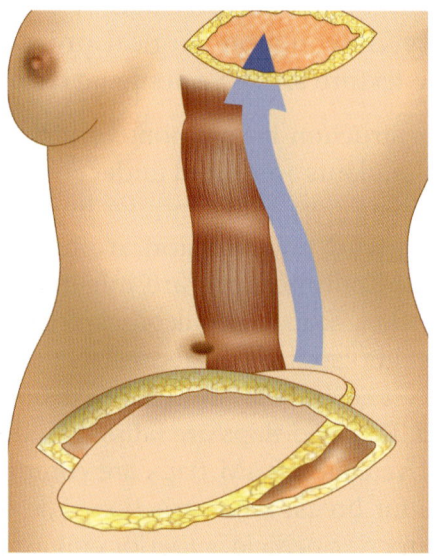

Fig. 3.1: TRAM flap

superior gluteal artery perforator flap and lateral septal gluteal artery perforator flap and free flap transfers from contralateral side.

Breast reconstruction using silicon gel implant under pectoralis major muscle is combined with prior tissue expansion using expandable saline prosthesis. Tissue expansion is used with breast prosthesis for breast reconstruction after mastectomy or breast equalisation for congenital breast asymmetry and tubular breast deformity.

Gigantomastia, excessive breast hypertrophy defined macromastia requiring surgical reduction of 1500 g of breast tissue. Reduction mammoplasty was performed and applied to extremely large volume breast reduction.[3]

Reduction mammoplasty is performed in women who are considered obese. Reduction mammoplasty is to reduce breast size while maintaining aesthetics and function. Earliest reduction was credited to Thorek. Earlier techniques used horizontal pedicles, vertical pedicles improved tissue perfusion. Nipple sensation is maintained for both superior and inferior pedicles. Vertical mammoplasty uses superior pedicle gives longer lasting attractive shape but learning curve is steep. Complications are haematoma, skin necrosis and scar hypertrophy.

2492 patients studied have commonest complication is surgical site infection and concluded that reduction mammoplasty is safe surgical procedure.[4] Reduction mammoplasty is the commonest procedure performed by plastic surgeons.[5] Patients benefit from reduction in breast size and symptoms of back pain, neck pain are relieved.[5] Inferior pedicle pattern reduction mammoplasty are commonest used by 69% of surgeons.[6] Liposuction is useful for moderate sized breast.

Breast reconstruction is crucial step for treatment of breast cancer. Local glandular flaps are used to restore breast shape and volume. Two types of flaps are used, the pedicled myo-cutaneous latissimus dorsi flap and deep inferior epigastric perforator flap. Latissimus dorsi flap and is simple and reliable but requires breast prosthetic material to add volume to reconstruction. The deep inferior epigastric perforator (DIEP) flap allows reconstruction providing high quality of supple tissues[7] (Figs 3.2 to 3.4).

Breast reconstruction after mastectomy should be integrated part in therapeutic approach of patient with breast cancer. Breast implant is commonly used for reconstruction.[8]

Breast reconstruction following breast conserving surgery for centrally located breast cancer at early stage is satisfactory for the aesthetic result and clinical efficacy and deserves further clinical application.

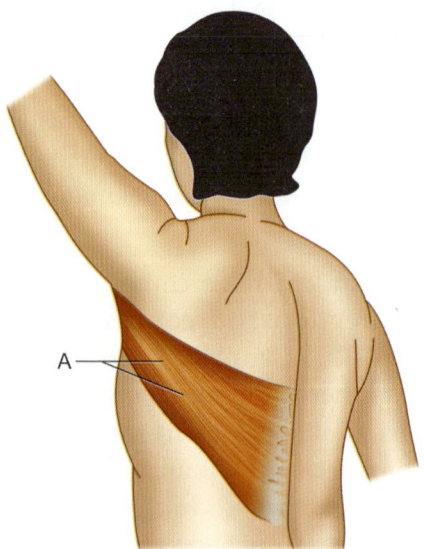

Fig. 3.2

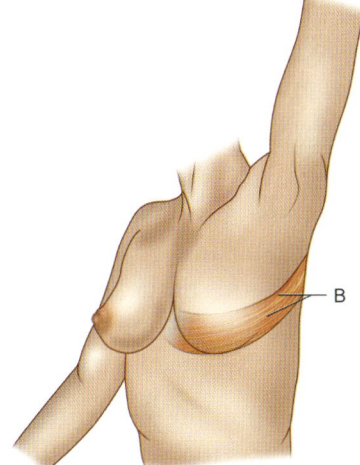

B

Fig. 3.3

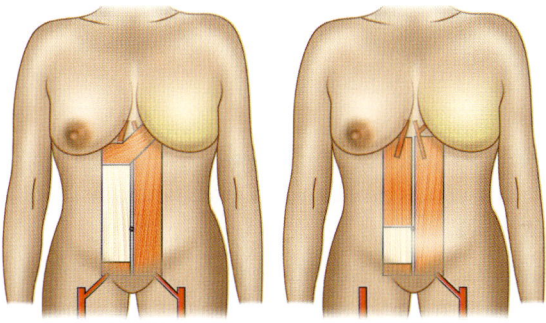

TRAM   Free TRAM

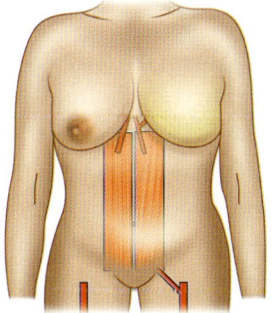

DIEP

Fig. 3.4

Reconstruction of nipple and areola are achieved by skin taken from inner thigh, labia and breast. Sagging caused by pregnancy, aging and weight loss mastopexy, breast lift operations are done. Nipple position elevated by appropriate skin excision.

Lipomodelling offers additional tool to refine breast reconstruction surgery. Starting from deeper layers to superficial layers in subcutaneous tissue. This study demonstrates that large volumes of fat that could be injected for sculture optimization and reshaping reconstructive breasts.[9]

Fat grafting called lipofilling or fat transfer where fat is taken from abdomen, buttocks is purified and layered to create desired shape. Reconstructive surgeons are using nerve regeneration procedure which enables tissue transplanted from abdomen for breast reconstruction to have breast reconstruction.

References

1. Veber M, Mojallal A. Breast reconstruction using muscle sparing latissimus dorsi and fat grafting. Ann Thir Plast Esthet 2012 April 11.

2. Beltese S, Gailloud Mathheir MC, Raffoul W, et al. Breast augmentation indications, types of prosthesis, surgical techniques, complications, results Dev Med Sisse Romande 1999 Sept;119(9): 729–37.

3. De George BR, Colen DL, Miricili AF, et al. Reduction mammoplasty operative techniques for improved outcomes in treatment of gigantomastia. Eplasty 2013 Oct 18;13:54.

4. Gust MJ, Smelona JT, Persing JS, et al. The impact of body mass index on reduction mammoplasty. A multicentre analysis of 2492 patients. Aesthetic Surg J 2013 Nov 8.

5. Kalliainen LK. ASPS health policy committee. ASPS clinical practice guideline summary on reduction mammoplasty. Plast Eeconstr Surg 2012;130(4):785–9.

6. Okara SA, Barone C, Bohnenblust M, et al. Breast reduction trends among plastic surgeons, a national survey. Plast Reconst Surg 2008;122(5):1312–20.

7. Berthe JV. Workhouse flaps for breast reconstruction. Rev Med Brux 2006 Sep;34(4):271–7.

8. Van Geertryden J. Breast reconstruction with implant. Rev Med Brux 2013 Sept;34(4):265–70.

9. Divido D, Demartene N, Clavien PA. Classification of surgical complications, a new proposal with evaluation in cohort of 6336 patients and results of survey. Ann Surg 2004;210:205–13.

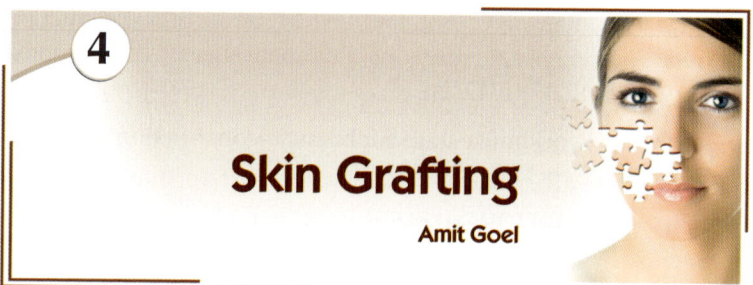

4

Skin Grafting

Amit Goel

Skin is the largest and most complex organ of the body. Its function includes protection against noxious agents, solar radiation, infections and thermal regulation. Dermis is 20 times thicker than epidermis. Skin is thickest over soles and thinnest over eyelids. During rest blood flow in skin is 15–20 ml/100 g/min and at full vascular dilatation it is 90 ml/min.

Bunger in 1823 was first to report successful skin grafting operation.[1] Grafts are biological dressing used for covering cutaneous defects and protecting the deeper structures from physical and chemical injuries. Grafted tissue becomes source of growth factor and interleukins which stimulate phase of repair. Skin graft is defined as piece of skin that has been separated from one part of body (donor area) and transplanted to another part of body (recipient site). Skin graft is segment of dermis and epidermis that has been removed from its blood supply and donor site.

The recipient surface undergoes plasmatic phase imbibition and layers of fibrin forms biological glue binding the graft to recipient and protecting from infection. This phase lasts 24–48 hours. The next phase is inosculation. There is capillary growth phase (revascularisation). There is activation and proliferation of keratinocytes during the phase of graft healing. Epidermal keratinocytes undergo mitosis and epidermis increases by seven to eight fold. Donor site heals by secondary intention. Process of epithelisation continues till complete area covered with skin. Inosculation and growth of blood vessels lasts from 4th to 7th day. If the bacterial count of recipient site is 105 bact/g and infection of streptococci, staphylococci, graft will not take up. Maturation of skin grafts occurs when there is contraction of graft due to myofibroblasts and contractile proteins.

Phase 1:0–48 hours—plasmatic imbibitions—diffusion of nutrition from recipient.

Phase 2: Inosculation—vessels in graft connect with those in recipient bed

Phase 3: Neovascular ingrowth—graft revascularized by new vessels **4–7 days**.

Management of Burns

- Remove from source of injury
- Airway, ventilation
- Wound care
- Decrease pain by analgesics
- Transport of patient
- Resuscitation

    Parkland formula: 4 ml X% burn X per kg body wt.

    This calculates fluid requirement in 1st 24 hours.

    Antibiotics used for dressing are silver sulphadiazine, silver nitrate, Mafenide is useful against Pseudomonas, Enterococcus.

    Daikin solution (0.25% sodium hypochlorite) is used for storage of grafts. Early excision and grafting is treatment of choice. Deep burns heal with grafting.

Types of Skin Grafts

- Split thickness—thin split, intermediate, thick
- Full thickness
- Tissue cultured

Split thickness skin grafts consist of epidermis and part of dermis. Depending on thickness, they are classified:

Thin: 0.006–0.012 inches thick.

Intermediate: 0.012–0.018 inches thick.

Thick: 0.018–0.030 inches thick.

Split thickness graft could be stored in Hank's solution containing plasma and neomycin in 4° for 21 days. Split thickness graft consists of obtaining STSG consisting of epidermis and part of dermis from selected donor site and grafted on recipient site. Equipment includes humby knife and bard parker handle (Fig. 4.1).

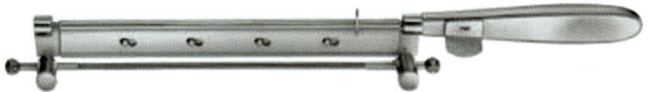

Fig. 4.1: Grafting knife

Full thickness grafts consist of epidermis and full thickness of dermis without subcutaneous fat layer. Full thickness skin grafts are preferred over split thickness skin grafts at sites like face.

A full thickness graft includes complete dermis where a split thickness graft comprises a varying amount of dermis. The thicker is the dermal component, closer to normal are characteristics of graft. During healing the graft receives nutrition and oxygen from interstitial fluid of wound. During the following weak new blood vessels joining with capillaries of graft start growing from wound. The skin graft donor site heals by epithelization from edges of the site. Local flaps are used in scalp reconstruction since they provide healthy, stable, hair bearing tissue and require short healing time for patients.[2] Culture media instead of saline, Hartmann solution should be used for temporary storage of split skin graft at 4°C. Graft should be meshed to expand the area of coverage. Stored meshed graft should be used within 7 days.[3]

Early tangential excision of nonviable burn tissue followed by immediate skin grafting with allograft has resulted in improvement of burn patient. Split thickness dermal grafts were grafted and forms new source of grafting tool for extensive deep partial and full thickness burns.[4]

Recipient area for grafting is judged by clinical appearance and bacterial count. Presence of beta haemolytic streptococci is contraindication for grafting. Donor site should be shaved. Grafts could be harvested with skin grafting knife which is pressed against thigh and with to and fro motion the knife moves forward. Blade has been set at predetermined depth, thickness of graft is influenced by pressure applied to skin. Graft should be meshed to expand it. Meshing device meshes the graft. A ratio of 1.5 : 1 provides minimal expansion but improves ability of graft. Ratio of 6 : 1 could be used for extensive burns. Skin grafting could be stored for 2 weeks at 4°C. Graft is placed over the recipient site and sutured. A dressing protects the graft.

Full thickness grafts are used to correct facial deformities. Postauricular sulcus, supraclavicular and infraclavicular regions are donor sites for full thickness grafts.

Composite grafts consist of epidermis and full thickness of dermis with subcutaneous fat. They contain skin, fat and underlying cartilage from donar site for auricle and nasal defects.

Skin substitutes are cultured autologous, allogus grafts. They are composed of epidermis elements, dermal elements. They are biological dressing and stimulate healing.

Cultured epidermal autografts consist of sheets of confluence tissues and keratinocytes. Skin samples are processed through cultures. 1 cm^2 skin could be expanded.

Free skin grafts is detached from body temporarily and transferred from donor to recipient site.

Cadaveric allografts derived from human cadaveric skin. After removing epidermis dermal cells are processed to produce nonantigenic acellular dermis.

Neonatal allografts derive from neonatal penile foreskin are harvested either on nylon, vicryl mesh. These fibroblasts secrete factors that produce neodermis.

Collagen grafts have chondrate sulphate that are used to produce dermal analogues.

Bilayered grafts are skin substitutes containing epidermal and dermal elements. They are derived from allogenic human keratinocytes. This bilayered graft provides skin covering to large skin defects.

- Dermal substitutes: Mesencymal cells
- Epithelial grafts: Full thickness
- Biological dressings: Keratinocytes, fibroblasts
- New technologies used for improving quantity and quality of skin grafting. Integra is dermal substitute with silicon cover. Grafting this on clean wound enhances replaced skin. Cultured epithelial autografts used for resurfacing extensive burns should be considered.

FLAPS

Flaps are used to transfer full thickness skin from one site to another.

Flaps are classified as:
- Local flaps—advancement, pivot, interpolation
- Distant flaps—cross leg, free flap

Flaps by location

Rhomboid—provides local cover (Fig. 4.2).

Pedicled—allows flap brought from distant site.

Free flap—microsurgery required for reconstruction.

Double transposition flap or Z plasty interchanges the position of two skin flaps on either side of incision or scar and is undertaken for reposition of distorted structures or scars and correct linear contractures. Z plasty is effective means of lengthening scars and consists of two triangular random pattern skin flaps raised next to one another on the area to be lengthened. Incision forms a Z and the change of axis of tissue tension allows lengthening of scar (Fig. 4.3).

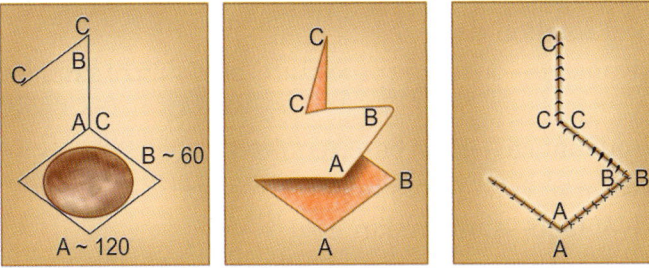

Fig. 4.2: Rhomboid flap

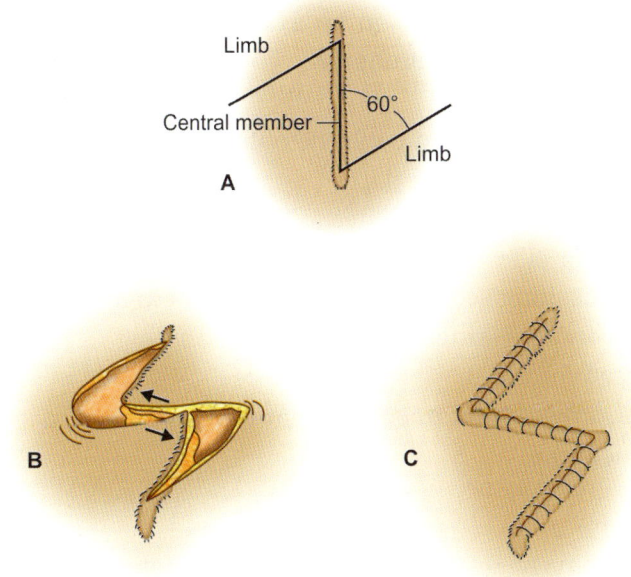

Fig. 4.3: Z plasty

Free Graft

Advantage—one stage procedure

Disadvantage—suitable for small areas

Tube pedicle

Advantage—could be swung anywhere

Disadvantage—limited length relative to width, prolonged immobilization

Local rotation flaps

Advantage—one stage procedure, uses skin of similar quality

Disadvantage—long base required

Cross transfers—cross finger, cross leg

Advantage—similar skin

Disadvantage—requires immobilization of healthy limb, digit

Newer techniques

Vascular pedicle flap

This is a flap based on an axial artery, temporal artery, branch of internal mammary

Advantages

Large areas of skin could be obtained

Small base for long flap

Free vascular flap

Area of skin detached with its supplying vessels which are reanastomosed to vessels in recipient area

Advantage—single stage procedure

Disadvantages

Requires skilled microvascular surgery

Thick flap

Skin Creams

Photodamage results from long-term deleterious effects of sun exposure characterised by coarse and fine wrinkling, mottled pigmented changes, textural roughness and telangiectasias. Topical *trans*-retinoic acid are used to treat acne vulgaris, photodamaged skin and hyperpigmentation. Adapalene derivative of naphthoic acid 0.1% gel cream improves skin irritation and acne. Sunscreens should be used to prevent photodamage and applied 2 mg/cm². Common antioxidants for healthy skin are vitamins A, C, E, coenzyme, alpha hydroxyl acid, green tea, polyphenols, selenium and zinc.

Multiple skin lightening agents available are hydroquinone inhibitor of tyrosinase combines with tretinoin, glycolic acid. Combination of hydroquinone 4%, tretinoin 0.05% and flucidone 0.01% have better efficacy.

References

1. Haben DJ, Barvchin A, Mahler D. On history of free skin graft. Ann Plast Surg 1982;(9):242–6.
2. Zayako Y, Staneo A, Mihailou H, et al. Application of local axial flaps to scalp reconstruction, Arch Plast Surg 2013 Sept; 40(5):564–9.
3. Li Z, Overend C, Maitz P, et al. Quality evaluation of meshed split thickness, skin grafts stored at 4°C in isotonic solutions and nutrient media by cell cultures. Burns 2012;38(6):899–907.
4. Application of split thickness dermal grafts in deep partial and full thickness burns, a new source of autoskin grafting. J Burn Care Res 2012 May–Jun; 33(3):94–100.

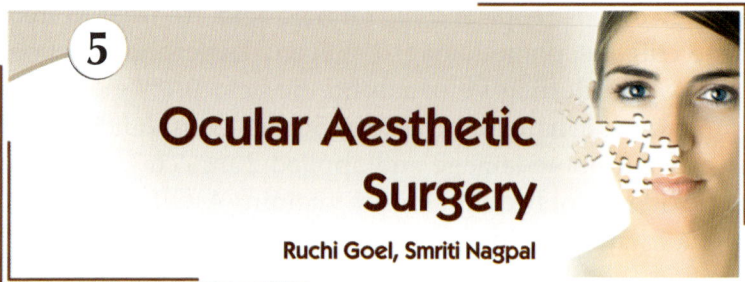

Ocular Aesthetic Surgery

Ruchi Goel, Smriti Nagpal

Cosmetic surgery is no longer a domain of plastic surgeons as it is now being practiced by practitioners in other disciplines.[1] According to the definition adopted by the American Medical Association (AMA) in 1989 'Cosmetic surgery is performed to reshape normal structures of the body to improve the patient's appearance and self esteem'.[2] It differs from reconstructive surgery which deals with abnormal structures of the body. The distinction from reconstructive surgery is important because our health care system recognizes the medical necessity of reconstructive surgery and insurance is willing to pay for it unlike cosmetic surgery. However, superior visual field interference due to ptosis of eyelid margin, excess hanging skin and lower lid laxity causing significant tearing are included under medical insurance.

FACIAL AESTHETICS

The face can be divided into three sections:

Part	Boundary	Parts
Upper third	Lies above the lateral canthal angle	Forehead, eyebrows and upper eyelids
Middle third/ Midface	Lies between lateral canthal angle and top of nasolabial fold	Lateral canthal tendon, medial canthal tendon, skin, fat, orbicularis oculi muscle of lower lid, the

(Contd.)

Part	Boundary	Parts (Contd.)
		suborbicularis oculi fat (SOOF) pad, the malar fat pad, orbitomalar ligament, orbital septum, origin of zygomaticus major and minor muscles and levator labii superioris
Lower third	Lies below the nasolabial fold	Structures below nasolabial fold

BLEPHAROPLASTY

Blepharoplasty in the contemporary usage refers to excision of excessive eyelid skin, with or without the excision of orbital fat for either functional or cosmetic indications.

A complete general medical and ocular history is obtained to rule out thyroid eye disease or other inflammatory diseases which may be responsible for abrupt changes in eyelid tissues. It is also important to diagnose a patient of bleeding disorders and dry eye. Dry eye may get exacerbated following surgery leaving the patient unhappier. With the help of photographs, the specific anatomic areas of concern and possible surgical solutions are discussed with the patient. A certain subset of patients suffering from body dysmorphic disorder (BDD) or dysmorphophobia may fixate on an imagined defect in appearance.[3] They may become distraught after surgery.[4] Individuals with relatively prominent globe and shallow orbit (negative vector orbit) need to be informed about the possibility of postoperative lid retraction.[5]

A thorough inspection of the periorbital and midface structures is fundamental and includes:
• Prominences of the supraorbital rim
• Malar hypoplasia

- Ptosis of the midface region
- Festoons
- Nasojugal depression
- Diamond shaped depression over the infraorbital foramen
- Brow position
- Forehead rhytids and frontalis muscle activity
- Glabellar lines

The functional indications for upper and lower eyelid blepharoplasty are as follows:[6]

1. Mechanical

- Dermatochalasis
- Epiblepharon
- Entropion

2. Inflammatory

- Graves' ophthalmopathy
- Blepharochalasis
- Floppy eyelid syndrome

3. Traumatic

- Contralateral orbital fracture with enophthalmos.
- After skin grafting for eyelid tissue or eyelid reconstruction.

Blepharoplasty may need to be combined with adjunctive procedures such as browplasty, ptosis repair, lateral canthoplasty, laser or chemical rejuvenation, midface lift or rhytidectomy.

Recently, there has been a shift towards fat repositioning. This technique however has been associated with lower eyelid retraction[7] and double vision. Also, sutured fat may predispose to focal necrosis, granuloma formation and scarring.

Repositioning of fat over the inferior orbital rim has been described to improve the soft tissue volume deficit that occurs in the upper cheek. Chemosis, hardening of transposed fat due to scarring and granuloma formation have been reported. Prolapsing the fat may cause motility disturbances due to incarceration of fibrovascular orbital septa that communicate with the extraocular muscles and lower eyelids.[8]

Upper Lid Blepharoplasty

The upper lid crease is marked 10 mm superior to the central eyelid margin in women and 7–8 mm in men. The medial extent of the incision should lie 5 mm superior to the superior punctum and lateral extent at least 5 mm superior to the lateral canthus. If required, the lateral end can be extended ~1.5 cm lateral to the lateral canthus and angled slightly superiorly. The amount of skin to be excised is determined (the distance between the inferior brow and superior incision line should be ~10–12 mm).

2–4 ml of infiltrative anaesthesia using 2% lidocaine with 1 : 100000 epinephrine is given subcutaneously. The skin-muscle excision may be combined with gentle fat excision followed by closure of skin. No traction is to be made on the fatty tissue to avoid injury to the deep vasculature (Fig. 5.1).

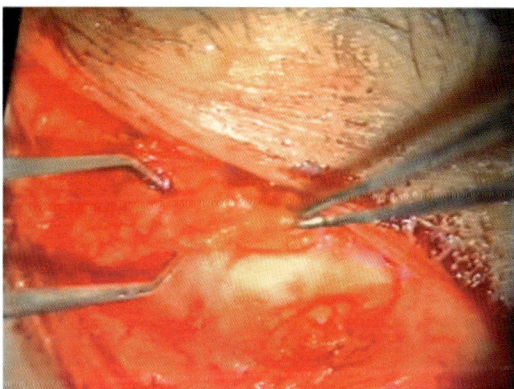

Fig. 5.1: The middle fat pad expose in the upper lid

Lower Lid Blepharoplasty

The lower lid blepharoplasty can be performed via a transcutaneous or transconjunctival approach.[9, 10] The transcutaneous approach allows direct access to manage orbicularis hypertrophy or excessive skin at the time of fat excision. The transconjunctival route has the merits of absence of visible scar, lesser chances of injury to orbital septum and direct access to lower eyelid fat pads (Figs 5.2 and 5.3).

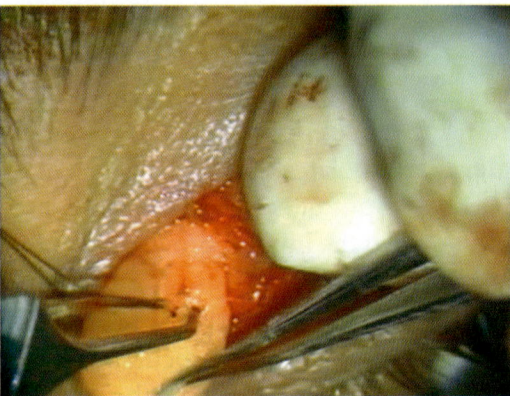

Fig. 5.2: Anterior approach in lower lid blepharoplasty with medial fat pad exposed

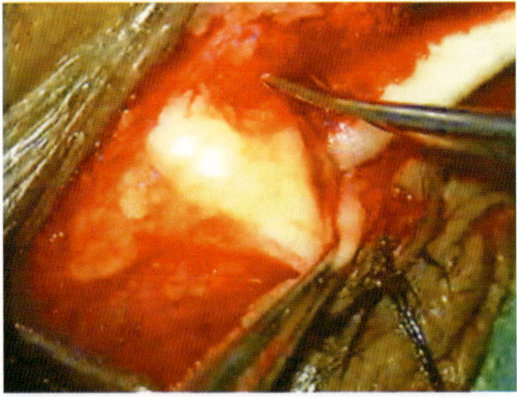

Fig. 5.3: The medial fat pad excised carefully to avoid damage to inferior oblique which lies between the central and medial fat pads

Transconjunctival Approach[11]

After local infiltrative anaesthesia, the conjunctiva and retractors are incised 5 mm inferior to the border of tarsal plate to approach orbital fat pads which are debulked in a graded fashion. After a judicious fat excision, the conjunctiva and lower lid retractors may be sutured with 6–0 absorbable sutures or left to close spontaneously.

The tear trough deformity correction requires release of ligamentous structures and orbicularis (of which the tear trough is composed) as well as fat transposition or fat grafting.[12]

Transcutaneous Technique

An infraciliary incision is placed 2 mm below the lash line, along the inferior lid, carried out 5–10 mm temporally past the lateral canthal angle and a subcutaneous dissection for 4 mm is carried out to reach inferior edge of the tarsal plate.

The orbicularis is incised and dissection of myocutaneous flap is carried out till the inferior orbital rim. The orbital septum is incised and fat pads are dissected and debulked or transposed. The myocutaneous flap is redraped into its anatomic position, and excess skin and orbicularis are excised.

Lower eyelid laxity if present is treated by lateral tarsal strip procedure, lateral canthoplasty, full thickness wedge resection, lateral canthal plication or pexy and retinaculum suspension procedures.[13]

Schiller has proposed a technique of carbon dioxide laser lysis of the orbicularis retaining ligament and the orbicularis oculi insertion into the maxilla to release the tethering of the lower lid and cheek and allow recontouring of the lid cheek junction in an extended transcutaneous lower blepharoplasty.[14]

The Midface Lift

Midface ptosis is manifested by pronounced nasojugal groove defined inferiorly by the leading edge of the ptotic malar fat pad and superiorly by lower eyelid fullness from pseudoherniated orbital fat.

Various approaches have been used for midface elevation, namely lateral, superolateral, superotemporal coronal/ temple incision, endoscopic coronocanthoplasty, extended infraciliary incision, etc. However, a lateral or superolateral pull results in an unnatural vector of lift because the midface soft tissue falls more in a vertical vector than in an inferior medial direction. Vertical elevation requires fixating mobilized suborbicularis oculi fat and midface soft tissues to the diaphanous inferior orbital arcus marginalis and orbital rim periosteal tissues. But the arcus marginalis lacks the strength to hold the sutures. Also, vertical lift does not address the involutional loss of the bone projection at the orbital rim and malar face. To compensate for the above, hand carved reinforced sheets of expanded polytetrafluoro-ethylene (ePTFE) have been used.[15]

The implant is anchored to the bone using titanium screws and the advanced midface tissues are securely sutured to the ePTFE implant at the orbital rim. Another approach to midface rejuvenation combines the use of percutaneous suture suspension technique and fat autografting.[16, 17]

Brow Lift

The brow lies in the upper third of face extending from the brow to the hairline. The brow should lie at the level of orbital rim. The male brow tends to be more horizontal whereas the female brow arches along its course over the orbital rim.[18]

Eyebrow ptosis results from gravitational descent and involutional changes in the deep supporting structures of the forehead. The eyebrow ptosis contributes to dermato-chalasia and temporal hooding of the eyes which results in contraction of the peripheral visual fields. Upper lid blepharoplasty can itself accentuate the tendency of the brow to move down.[19] The procedures used to correct brow ptosis are browpexy, direct brow lift, a midforehead lift, a pretrichial forehead lift, a coronal forehead lift and an endoscopic midforehead elevation.

DIRECT BROWPEXY

Direct browpexy is performed for mild to moderate brow ptosis. Through a blepharoplasty incision, the dissection is extended superiorly, the brow fat is identified and the deep dermal tissues are affixed to the periosteum with one to three permanent sutures.

Disadvantages include decreased brow mobility, regression of the procedure and bleeding.

Direct Brow Lift (Browplasty)

It involves excision of skin above the brow hairs and results in elevation of the eyebrow under the area of skin excision. It is best suited to individuals who are willing to tolerate some visible scarring.[20]

Midforehead Browplasty

It involves a direct excision of forehead skin above the brows and is suited for patients with deep forehead creases.

Coronal Forehead Elevation

The incision across the scalp and into the temporal areas elevates the brow, temporal hooding and reduces rhytids in the lateral canthal area (crow's feet). Patients with a receding hairline are not good candidates for the procedure.

The Pretrichial Forehead Lift

The incision is placed in the hairline at the junction of the hair bearing and non-hair bearing skin. The skin anterior to the incision is excised thereby shortening the forehead and advancing the hairline forward.

Endoscopic Midforehead Elevation

This involves small, hidden incisions and minimal to no excision of the skin. It can be performed in patients with hair recession pattern.[21] Most techniques involve five small incisions—central sagittal 0.5–1 cm behind the hairline, 2 cm in length anteroposteriorly;[2] similar incisions 3–4 cm on either side of the midline incision behind the hairline and one incision is placed in each temporal hair tuft.

After local anaesthesia, appropriate dissection is carried out; the fibers of procerus and corrugators are identified, weakened or excised. The central and temporal flaps are elevated and fixated to the outer table of the cranium. In the temporal pocket, permanent fixation sutures are used to elevate the mobile temporal parietal fascia and attach them to the fascia of temporalis muscle.

The patient satisfaction is high and postoperative down time is less than in procedures involving larger amounts of skin excision.[22]

Conclusion

Cosmetic surgery and the adjunctive office procedures now occupy an important position in the mainstream. These procedures attempt to restore the aging individual to a youthful configuration so as to provide a greater level of self confidence. Amongst the various techniques practiced, patient selection, facial analysis of aging changes, patient desires and expectations and surgical experience determine the optimal method for each patient.

Expectations about results of these interventions run high, despite all attempts to encourage realism, but in majority of cases, results at least approximate expectation.

References

1. Tanna N, Lesavoy MA, Kawamoto HK, et al. Experiential learning in aesthetic surgery training: A quantitative comparison among surgical subspecialties. Plast Reconstr Surg. 2012 Mar;129(3):528e–34.

2. Nahai F. What is aesthetic surgery, anyway? Aesthetic Surgery Journal 2010; 30(6):874–5.

3. Mawn LA, Jordan DR. Dysmorphophobia: A distorted perception of one's self appearance. Ophthal Plast Reconstr Surg 1998;14:446–50.

4. Rohrich RJ. The who, what, when and why of cosmetic surgery: Do our patients need a preoperative psychiatric evaluation? Plast Reconstr Surg 2000;106:1605–7.

5. Hirmand H, Codner MA, McCord CD, et al. Prominent eye: Operative management in lower lid and midfacial rejuvenation and morphologic classification system. Plast Reconstr Surg 2002;110:620–34.

6. American Academy of Ophthalmology: Functional indications for upper and lower lid blepharoplasty. Ophthalmology 1995; 102:693.

7. Goldberg RA, Yuen VH. Restricted ocular movements following lower eyelid fat repositioning. Plast Reconstr Surg 2002;110:302–5.

8. Pessa JE. A logarithm of facial aging:verification of Lambro's theory by three-dimensional stereolithography, with reference to the pathogenesis of midfacial aging, scleral show and lateral suborbital trough deformity. Plast Reconstr Surg 2000; 106:479–88.

9. Perkins SW, Batnjii RK. Rejuvenation of the lower eyelid complex. Facial Plast Surg 2005;21:279–85.

10. Lee AS, Thomas JR. Lower lid blepharoplasty and canthal surgery. Facial Plast Surg Clin North Am 2005;13:541–51.

11. Camiranand A, Doucet J, Harris J. Eyelid aging: The historical evolution of its management. Aesthetic Plast Surg 2005; 29:65–73.

12. Stutman RL, Codner MA. Tear trough deformity: Review of anatomy and treatment options. Aesthetic Surg J. 2012 May 1; 32(4):426–40.

13. Holck DEE, Foster JA, Kalwerisky K. Lower eyelid blepharoplasty and midface elevation surgery. In: Albert Jakobiec's principles and Practice of Ophthalmology, 3rd edition. Saunders Elsevier 2008, 3471–82.

14. Schiller JD. Lysis of the orbicularis retaining ligament and orbicularis oculi insertion: A powerful modality for lower eyelid and cheek reconstruction. Plast Reconstr Surg 2012 Apr; 129(4):692e–700.

15. Steinsapir KD. Aesthetic and restorative midface lifting with hand carved, expanded polytetrafluoroethylene orbital rim implants. Plast Reconstr Surg 2003;111:1727–37.

16. Keller GS, Namazie A, Blackwell K, et al. Elevation of the malar fat pad with a percutaneous technique. Arch Facial Plastic Surg 2002;4:20–25.

17. Sasaki GH, Cohen AT. Meloplication of the malar fat pad by percutaneous cable suture technique for midface rejuvenation: Outcome study (392 cases, 6 years experience). Plast Reconstr Surg 2002;110:635–54.

18. Sullivan MJ. Brow and forehead aesthetics. Facial Plast Surg Clin North Am 1997;5:95–98.

19. Prado RB, Silva-Junior DE, Padovani CR, et al. Assessment of eyebrow position before and after upper eyelid blepharoplasty. Orbit 2012 May 9 [Epub ahead of print].

20. Booth AJ, Murray A, Tyers AG. The direct brow lift:Efficacy, complications and patient satisfaction. Br J Ophthalmol 2004; 88:688–91.

21. Steinsapir KD, Shorr N, Hoenig J, et al. The endoscopic forehead lift. Ophthal Plast Reconstr Surg 1998;14:107–18.

22. Puig CM, La Ferriere KA. A retrospective comparison of open and endoscopic brow lifts. Arch Facial Plast Surg 2002;4:221–5.

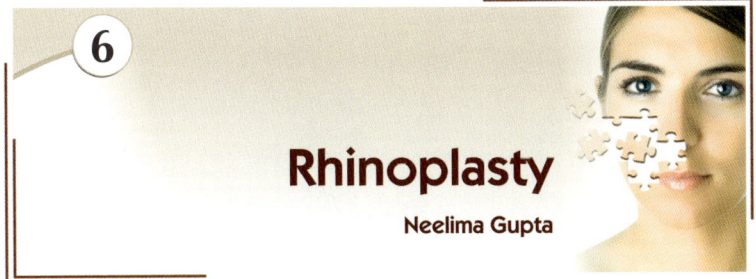

6

Rhinoplasty

Neelima Gupta

Nose is one of the very important part of the face contributing to its aesthetics. The "perfect nose" is dictated by the shape of the face, sex, ethnicity and symmetry with other parts of the face. Features which are generally considered to be contributing to a perfect nose are: a straight nasal dorsum, a narrow nasal tip, appropriate facial angles and nasal projection.

Rhinoplasty aims at modification or correction of the shape and contour of the nose keeping the proportion and facial angles in mind.

External nasal deformities are often associated with a disturbance of nasal function. Functional and aesthetic surgery of the nose usually involves a combined operation on the nasal septum and the external nose—septorhino-plasty.

The surgery is undertaken for deformities such as a prominent hump, a saddle nose, crooked nose and for tip deformities (Figs 6.1 and 6.2).

SURGICAL ANATOMY OF THE NOSE

The relevant surgical anatomy will be briefly discussed here. For detailed anatomy the readers are advised to follow a textbook, especially before embarking on this surgery.

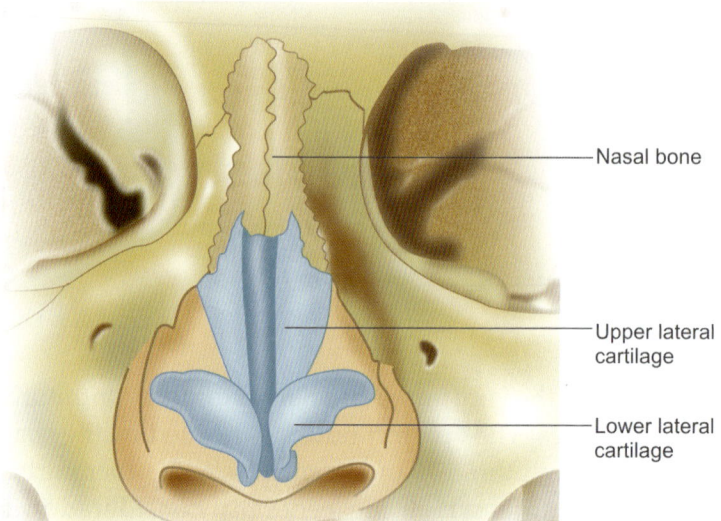

Fig. 6.1

Nasal bone

Upper lateral cartilage

Lower lateral cartilage

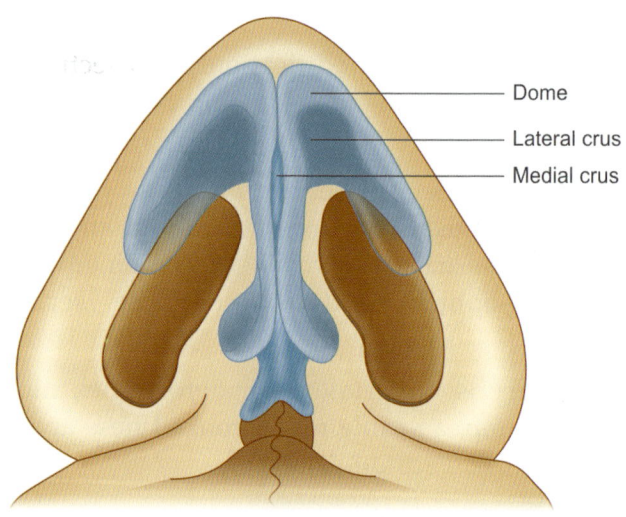

Fig. 6.2

Dome

Lateral crus

Medial crus

The nose can be divided into external skin and soft tissue, underlying framework (bony and cartilaginous), and ligamentous support. The osseocartilaginous nasal framework is comprised of three areas: the bony dorsum, the upper cartilaginous part and the lower cartilaginous part. The bony dorsum is constituted mainly by the nasal bones which articulate with the frontal process of the maxilla on either side. The upper edge of the upper lateral cartilages is attached to the undersurface of the lower edge of the nasal bones. Medially the upper lateral cartilages are continuous with the septal cartilage and laterally they are separated from the pyriform aperture by dense fibrous tissue. The two lower lateral cartilages consist of a medial crus, a lateral crus and a dome. The two medial crura are folded medially and contribute to formation of columella. The nasal tip is formed by the two domes as shown in Figs 6.3 and 6.4.

The columella is formed by the caudal end of the septum, the nasal spine and the medial crura of the lower lateral cartilages. The angle formed between the upper lip and the columella with its apex at the subnasale is the **nasolabial angle**. This is about 90–95° in the males and 100–110° for females. This angle contributes to the tip projection in lateral profile. These angles are shown in Fig. 6.5.

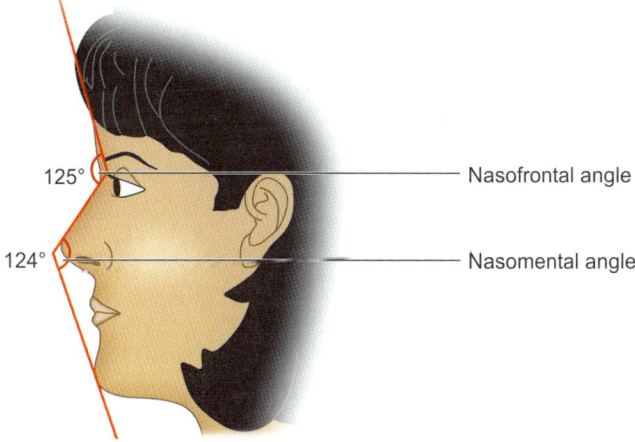

Fig. 6.3

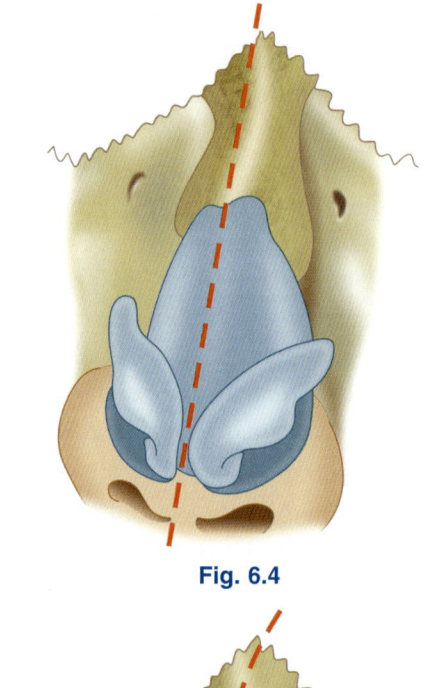

Fig. 6.4

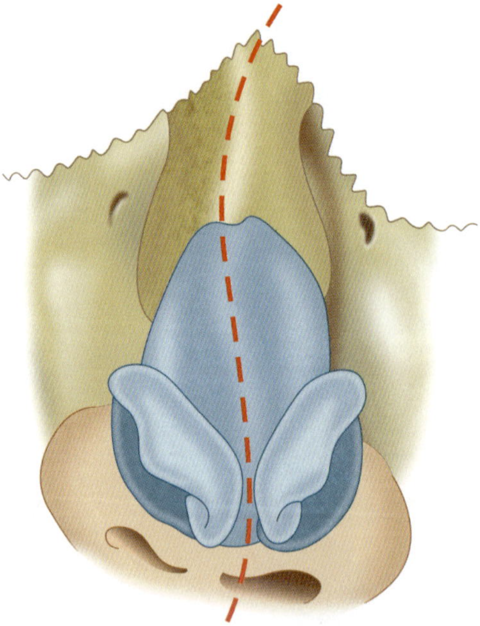

Fig. 6.5: S-shaped deviation

Another angle of the nose is the **nasofrontal angle**. It is the angle formed between the dorsum of the nose and the glabella. This angle is obtuse and ranges between 120 and 125° in profile.

Anaesthesia for Rhinoplasty

The surgery can be done under local or general anaesthesia. General anaesthesia is preferred in cases where osteotomies are required and in cases where graft needs to be harvested from iliac crest in cases of augmentation rhinoplasty. The pharyngeal pack is *in situ* to prevent any aspiration complications. Local anaesthesia may be used in co-operative adults where minor work is required on the nasal dorsum or only tip modification is required. The bleeding is less and the procedure is safer but co-operation required from the patient is more. Xylocaine sensitivity testing should be done preoperatively in all patients.

In case general anaesthesia is given, then the endotracheal tube should be preferably fixed in midline, to prevent distortion of the lip and the alar base of the nose. The administration of adrenaline saline is still recommended for facilitation of dissection.

If local anaesthesia is used then 2% xylocaine with adrenaline (1 : 1000), is used for infiltration. The infiltration is given in the

1. Infraorbital foramen region: The left hand is used to palpate the infraorbital margin and the anaesthetic is infiltrated in that region through a needle inserted 1 cm lateral to alar margin, directed superiorly.

2. Columellar base: The base of columella is infiltrated.

3. Dorsum of the nose: In this area it is important to anesthetize the infratrochlear (between the medial canthus and nasion) and the external nasal nerves (at

the lower edge of the nasal bones). Needle is inserted through the nasal cavity and local is injected along the dorsum of the nose. Care should be taken that the infiltration is not too much as it will impair the proper assessment of a preoperative depression or a hump on the dorsum of nose.

While the local is being injected it is important to keep a watch on the pulse rate and the blood pressure of the patient as sometimes due to rapid injection of the drug or due to accidental injection into a blood vessel, the vitals of the patient can get compromised. While operating the patient under local anaesthesia it is also important to keep a watch on the amount of blood trickling into the pharynx and the consciousness status of the patient.

Preoperative Assessment

Careful surgical planning is a prerequisite for rhinoplasty. A detailed analysis of the underlying anatomic cause of the deformity is essential to plan the course of surgery. Good preoperative photographs showing the frontal, lateral and basal profiles are a must before surgery. The nose must not only be looked at in isolation, but also with respect to the rest of the face, in order to create or preserve overall facial balance and harmony.

The patient needs to have a clear and realistic under-standing of the results achievable by surgery and the limita-tions of surgery. A psychiatric assessment preoperatively is in order if there is a mismatch between the complaints of the patient and the assessment of the surgeon with regard to the deformity. It is important also to assess the nasal skin texture. In patients with a thick skin corrections made in the cartilage or bone are not apparent while in patients with a thin skin minor irregularities or asymmetry are very much noticeable after closure.

Surgery is generally not undertaken before the age of 15 to 16 years because the septum and nasal bones may grow till that time and best results may not be achieved.

The aim is to give a natural appearance to the nose, maintain structural support of the dorsum and be conservative in resection of structures.

The front view is assessed first. Any asymmetry of the nasal dorsum or deviation is assessed by drawing a vertical line from the mid-glabella to the menton. The alar base and the tip are also assessed along with the curvilinear dorsal aesthetic lines.

The nose is assessed from the base, and the outline of the nasal base and the nostril is analyzed. The outline of the nasal base should describe an equilateral triangle with a lobule-to-nostril ratio of 1 : 2.

The lateral view is assessed for the nasofrontal angle, the nasolabial angle and the alar columellar relationship. Other deformities such as nasal hump and depression of nasal dorsum are also assessed on the lateral profile view.

Along with the external nose it is important to perform the intranasal examination to assess the nasal septum, turbinates and the nasal valve area. If nasal septum is deviated, the deviation is assessed and the surgical steps are planned accordingly.

Surgical Approaches

The nasal dorsum can be approached either through an endonasal (closed) or an external (open) approach.

The patient lies supine with his head end elevated about 20°. Proper top light along with surgeon head light is used. The nose, forehead and surrounding face area is prepared. When drapes are placed care is taken that the forehead and part of the eyes are left exposed. The hairs in the vestibule are clipped and the nasal cavities are cleaned.

Endonasal Approach

This approach is preferred when the correction is required mainly in the nasal dorsum such as in cases with hump nose or in crooked nose when osteotomies are indicated.

The endonasal incision is made in the skin of the vestibule. For minor deformities a hemitransfixion and intercartilaginous incision in one side of the nasal cavity is sufficient. In some cases where more modifications are required then bilateral intercartilaginous incisions with a transfixion incision is preferred. The transfixion incision divides the membranous septum anterior to the caudal septal margin. The intercartilaginous incisions are incisions made between the cephalic border of the lower lateral cartilage and the caudal border of the upper lateral cartilage (Fig. 6.6). This site is prominent inside the nasal cavities on inspection and can be gently visualized by putting some external pressure

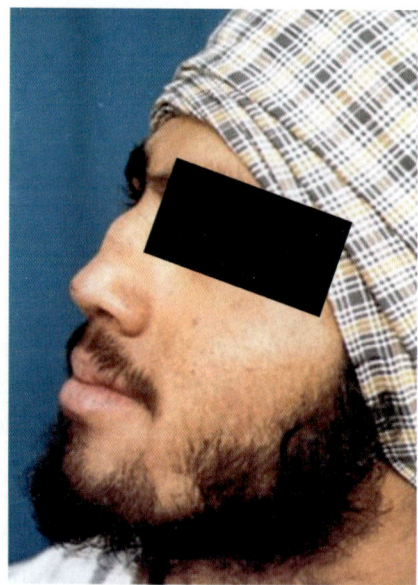

Fig. 6.6

on the upper lateral cartilage. The intercartilaginous incisions meet the transfixion incision and then the plane is formed above the perichondrium covering the upper lateral cartilages to visualize the nasal dorsum.

The soft tissues are elevated over the perichondrium and then under the periosteum, to reach the bony dorsum (Fig. 6.7). With this subperiosteal dissection the muscle is elevated with the flap and the dorsum is clearly visualized. The skin along with the flap is elevated using the Aufricht retractor.

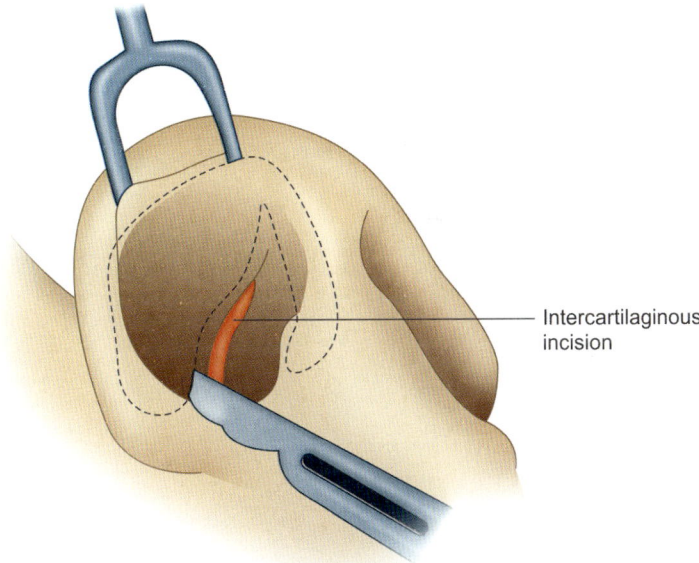

Intercartilaginous incision

Fig. 6.7

External Approach

The open approach is preferred by some surgeons because it provides a good exposure of the nasal framework, manipulation of the framework can be precise and under good vision, the grafts placed can be sutured so that extrusion or slippage decreases and complex tip modifications can be better addressed. It is a preferred approach in revision rhinoplasty. The disadvantage of this approach is the columellar scar.

For this approach, bilateral marginal incisions are given along the alar rim. These incisions are extended up to the middle of the caudal edge of the medial crura of the lower lateral cartilages and then combined to a horizontal or an inverted V incision in the mid-columella (Fig. 6.8). The skin of the nose is then dissected along the superior aspect of the cartilaginous vault and bony dorsum. This approach gives an excellent view of the nasal dorsum and cartilage modifications such as excision, suturing, insertion of spreader grafts and columellar strut placement, etc. can be done under vision. Care should be taken to protect the upper

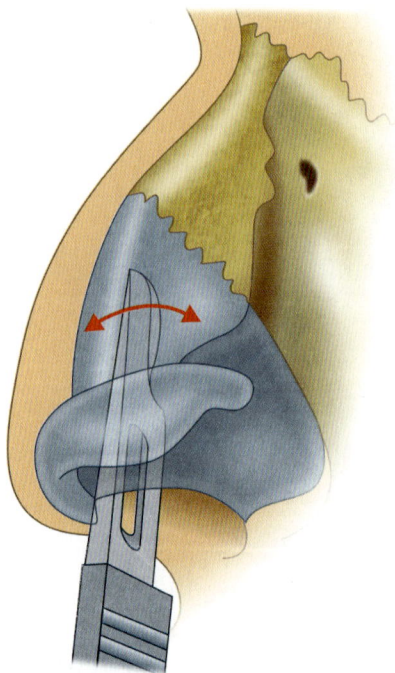

Fig. 6.8: Elevation of perichondrium

lateral cartilages and the dissection is done close to the perichondrium and periosteum. If any work needs to be done on the septum then it can be divided from the cartilages and then sutured later on.

After completion of the refinements, the marginal incisions are closed with chromic catgut. The columellar incision is sutured using prolene or fine silk sutures with careful approximation of the edges. With a good closure the scar is minimal and not visible.

HUMP REDUCTION

A hump can be bony, cartilaginous or combined bony and cartilaginous. The surgery involves reduction of the nasal hump, but the preoperative assessment should include assessment of the thickness of the skin, the amount of cartilaginous and bony hump, the width of the hump and most importantly the projection of the nasal tip. The hump should be removed above an imaginary line between the tip projection and the nasofrontal angle.

In very thin skins care has to be taken about trauma to the skin and also all irregularities after hump reduction need to be smoothened out because they will look unsightly once the skin is redraped over the dorsum. In patients with thick skin an undercorrection will lower the final effect after replacement of the flap so that should be kept in mind. The second complication which can arise is due to incomplete resection of the cartilaginous hump. Incomplete removal of cartilage from the supratip region leads to a "polly-beak deformity". In cases with a drooping tip the tip projection should be corrected and then the hump should be reduced accordingly because the patient may be having a "pseudohump" due to a ptotic or a drooping tip. If the hump is removed without correction of the tip projection, the nose will appear excessively long.

Surgical procedure: The dorsum of the nose is exposed using an endonasal or an external approach. The cartilaginous hump can be incised using a scissor or a knife. The bony hump can be removed using a rasp or a chisel. All soft tissue attachments should be severed before pulling out the removed part to prevent trauma. Any irregularities on inspection or palpation should be smoothened out. The dorsal profile is then assessed for the result.

After removal of the hump, the nasal dorsum in most cases becomes wide. To correct this deformity, narrowing of the nose using lateral osteotomies and debulking of excessive tissue along the upper lateral cartilages is desirable.

Osteotomies: Lateral osteotomies are used to narrow the lateral walls of the nose and also in cases where straightening of the nasal dorsum is required. Lateral osteotomy may need to be combined with a medial osteotomy in some cases or alternatively a curved lateral osteotomy can be done. An osteotome is the preferred instrument as it is less traumatic and leads to less bone dust and postoperative oedema. A 2–3 mm osteotome is used. It can be inserted intranasally through an incision just anterior to the attachment of the inferior turbinate at the edge of the pyriform aperture or through a stab incision externally. The intranasal incision is not combined with the intercartilaginous incision and may not be sutured later. The periosteum is elevated along the frontal process of maxilla and the osteotome is slowly advanced along the nasofacial groove with the right hand; the left hand being used to stabilize it and to protect the skin and soft tissues by maintaining the direction of the osteotome. The osteotomy is extended till the lower end of the frontal spine and care is taken to protect the medial canthal attachment (Fig. 6.9). If a curved osteotomy is planned the direction of the osteotome is curved medially to produce a green stick fracture in the nasal bones. Once osteotomy is done on both

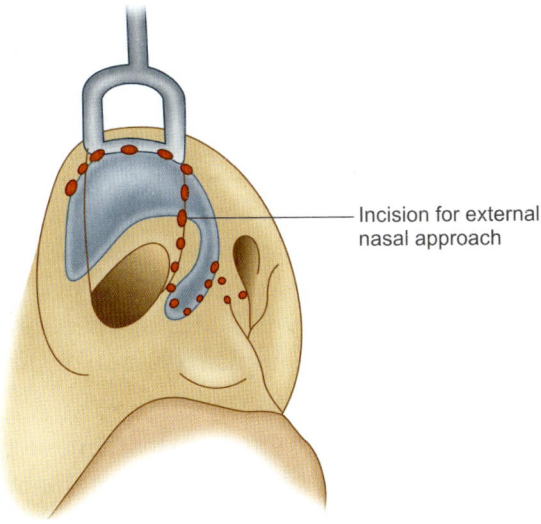

Incision for external nasal approach

Fig. 6.9

the sides the nasal bones and lateral nasal wall is gently mobilized, infractured and then adjusted in the proper position.

Medial osteotomy: In some cases if the lateral osteotomies have not been able to sufficiently mobilize the nasal bones then medial osteotomies may be needed. The osteotome is put at the lower end of the nasal bone, close to the nasal septum. The skin of the nasal vault is lifted up and the osteotome is advanced upwards, using taps of the mallet. On reaching the frontonasal suture, the osteotome is turned laterally and the nasal bones are outfractured. This mobilizes the framework of the nasal dorsum and then with the steady force of the right hand the surgeon narrows the nasal dorsum and straightens any deformity.

Complication: Apart from creating a polly-beak deformity, another complication is creating an "open-root deformity". After bony hump removal the nasal bridge is left open so lateral and medial osteotomies are required to infracture the nasal bones. If the lateral osteotomies are incomplete this open-roof deformity can persist.

CROOKED NOSE

The deviated nose or crooked nose is the condition when nasal dorsum is deviated from the median plane (Figs 6.10 and 6.11). It presents as a disturbance in alignment of the osseocartilaginous framework and apart from cosmetic problem patient may also complain of nasal obstruction due to septal displacement and deviation.

The management mostly entails osteotomies for the bony realignment and septal surgery for straightening of the cartilaginous framework. The approach used is mostly endonasal especially if mainly osteotomies are required with none or minimal tip work.

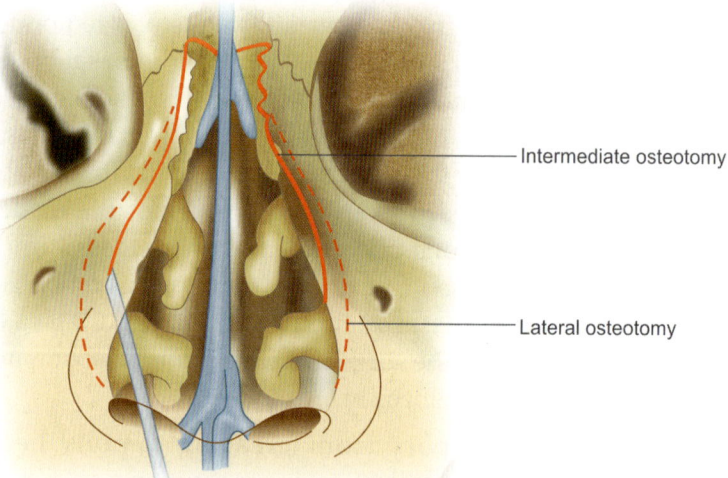

Intermediate osteotomy

Lateral osteotomy

Fig. 6.10

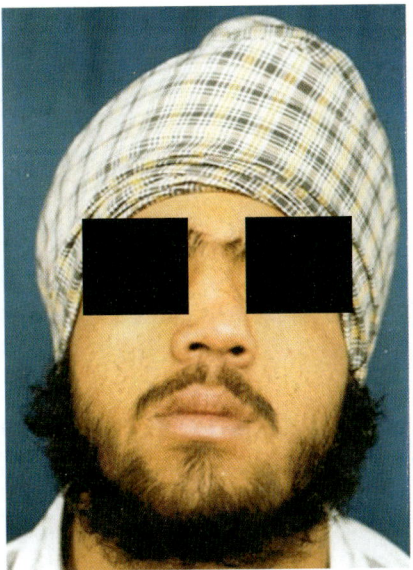

Fig. 6.11: Deviated nose

The patient is to be cautioned regarding the recurrence of the deviation because of the "memory effect" of the structures. The postoperative care in cases where osteotomies have been done includes keeping a plaster of Paris cast for at least 10 days after surgery; avoidance of any trauma to the nose and avoidance of manipulation by the patient. Figures 6.12 and 6.13 show the preoperative and postoperative profile of a patient with deviated nose.

SADDLE NOSE

This is a term given to a depressed nasal dorsum. A saddle nose is commonly a result of infected septal hematoma, nasal septal injury or sometimes due to chronic granulomatous conditions of the nose which lead to necrosis of the nasal septum.

Correction of the depression requires graft placement on the nasal dorsum and the procedure is referred to as augmentation rhinoplasty. Many options are available for

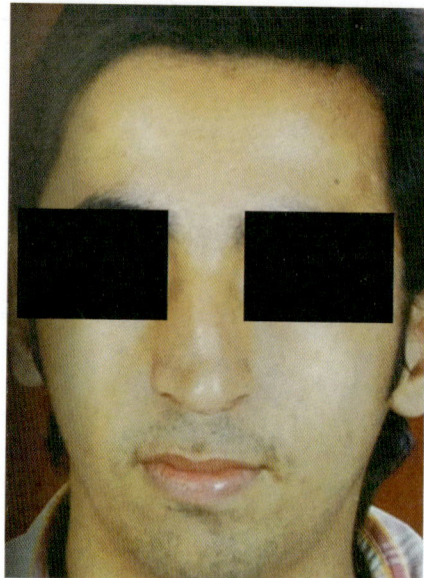

Fig. 6.12: Deviated nose—preoperative profile

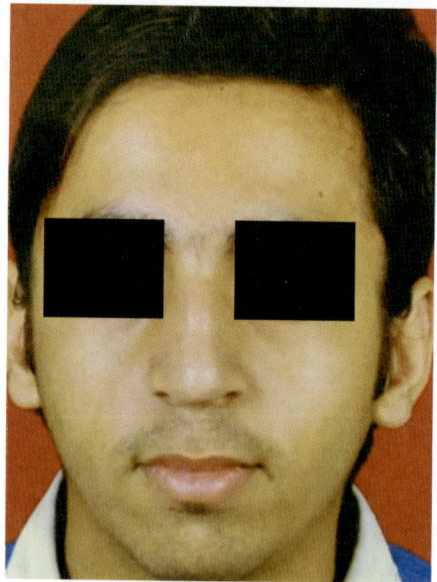

Fig. 6.13: Postoperative profile

this purpose and depending upon the degree and extent of the depression the graft can be chosen. For small depressions involving the cartilaginous dorsum, a cartilage graft is preferred. This graft is mostly harvested from the conchal cartilage of the pinna. If the saddle involves the cartilaginous and bony dorsum, then an iliac crest graft or costal cartilage graft needs to be used.

Often an external approach is preferred for augmentation rhinoplasty because the graft can be placed properly under vision and if need be suturing can be done. Also most of these cases require tip remodelling and columellar graft placement, which is easier using open approach. But the surgery can also be done using intercartilaginous incisions in an endonasal approach.

The conchal cartilage is most often used for nasal dorsum augmentation. It is harvested using a postural incision. The cartilage is identified and then removed along with the perichondrium on the posterior surface. A contour dressing is done to prevent blood collection and hematoma formation.

The complications of this procedure include displacement and extrusion of the graft. Extrusion is more common with alloplastic materials like silastic. Other complications include infection of the graft, necrosis of the skin overlying the graft (if the graft is too big or it has been fitted in a tight pocket) and resorption of the graft over a period of time. Figures 6.14 and 6.15 show preoperative and postoperative profile of a patient with depressed nose.

NASAL TIP RHINOPLASTY

The nasal tip is an integral part of the nose and gives a definition to the nose. But tip refinements require a lot of finesse and skill.

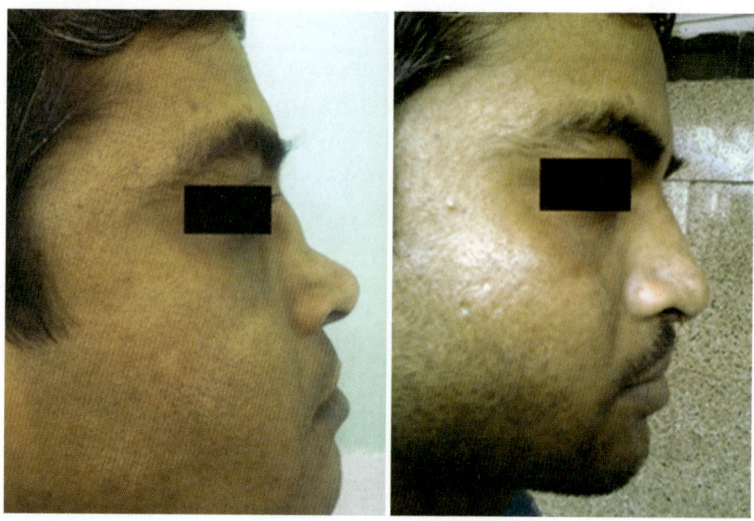

Figs 6.14 and 6.15: Depressed nose—preoperative and postoperative

One of the common cosmetic problems with the tip is the bulbous tip. This is mostly due to fullness of the cephalic aspect of the alar cartilages. This requires excision of part of the lateral crura of the lower lateral cartilages and interdermal sutures for the narrowing of the tip. This can be done using the external approach which provides excellent exposure of the cartilaginous vault or using the delivery flap technique which uses the marginal incisions.

Other deformity which may require attention is a bifid nasal tip. Increasing tip projection is often required along with hump removal in some patients. At times a condition of "alar-collapse" may be encountered. This is because of weak or medially convex lateral crura of the lower lateral cartilage which prolapse inwards on inspiration. This is corrected by placing a stabilizing graft in the alae.

Excessive removal of vestibule skin and lower lateral cartilages can lead to a "knock-kneed" tip deformity. This is more common in patients with thin skin and lax cartilages.

Closure of Incisions and Dressing

Whichever approach is used, before closure of the incisions, care needs to be taken that all fine refinements of the tip and cartilage reshaping has been done. The rough edges have been smoothened out and bone dust has been washed out. Any blood which is collected over the dorsum is squeezed out. The incisions are sutured using 3/0 or 4/0 chromic catgut sutures. Nasal cavities are packed lightly with soframycin soaked 1 cm ribbon gauze. This pack is to be removed after 48 hours. The skin is then draped over the dorsum using micropore strips which are placed horizontally, overlapping each other in half of their width; starting from the nasion to the supratip region. The tip is also covered using a vertical strip of micropore tape. These strips prevent postoperative hematoma formation and decrease postoperative ecchymosis. If osteotomies have been done then the nose will need to be splinted using plaster of Paris. This protects the nose from minor trauma, prevents movement of the nasal bones which have been mobilized with osteotomies and also prevents swelling. The measurement of the nose is taken using a paper template and then a six layered plaster of Paris bandage is cut in the same size and shape. This is fixed on the nose and once it dries it is fixed to the skin using leukoplast or dynaplast tapes. The tip of the nose is covered with a nasal gauze bolster for soakage of any blood. The bolster is taped separately to the skin so that it can be removed or changed if required without disturbing the rest of the dressing. The patients head is kept elevated in the postoperative recovery room to decrease soft tissue edema.

The splint is to be removed after 10 days. In between if it becomes too loose then it should be changed. When the splint and the micropore tapes are removed the removal is done gently and after lubrication so that there is no trauma to the healing tissues.

COMPLICATIONS OF RHINOPLASTY

Any major complications are rare after rhinoplasty.

One of the common complications is postoperative bleeding. The bleeding can be mostly controlled with packing of the nose. If bleeding can be localised the bleeding point can be cauterised.

Necrosis of the skin can occur if the graft pocket is very superficial or tight, or if the vascularity of the skin has been compromised.

Infection at the osteotomy sites is rare but occasionally it can occur. It responds to antibiotics.

Excess removal of tissues is the main cause of complications in rhinoplasty. Overzealous removal of hump, not maintaining an appropriate level of the septal cartilage and the upper lateral cartilages, improper infracturing of the nasal bones can all lead to worsening of the deformity in the postoperative period.

If the skin is too thin then any irregularities of the bone will be very unsightly. Inadequate rasping in these patients will lead to residual deformity. If the graft is not properly fitted in these patients then graft edges may also protrude out and look very unsightly.

The aim of the rhinoplastic surgeon should be to give as normal an appearance to the nose as possible with correction of the gross deformities.

References

1. Corrective Rhinoplasty by V. P. Sood. CBS Publishers and Distributors, New Delhi. First edition 1996.

2. ENT-Head and Neck surgery: Essential Procedures. G. Rettinger. EdsJuergenTheissing, Gerhard Rettinger, Jochen A. Werner. Georg ThiemeVerlag, Stuttgart, New York; 2011.

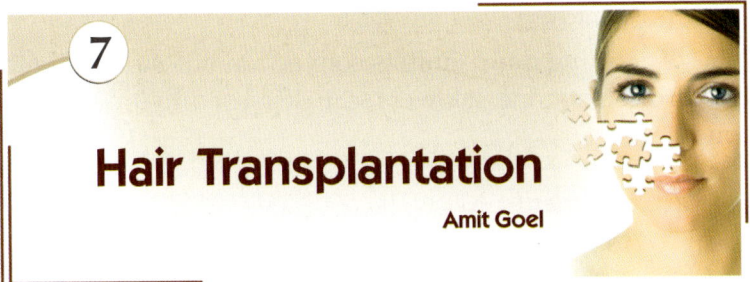

7

Hair Transplantation

Amit Goel

Shedding of hair is termed effluvium and resulting condition is called alopecia. Alopecia classified into noncicatricial alopecia having no clinical signs of tissue inflammation, scarring, atrophy of skin and cicatricial alopecia having evidence of tissue destruction. Inflammation, atrophy and scarring is apparent. Pattern hair loss is commonest type of progressive balding. It occurs through combined effect of genetic predisposition and action of androgen on scalp hair follicles. Male pattern hair loss varies from bitemporal recession to frontal and vertex thinning and along occipital and temporal margins. Male alopecia begins after puberty expressed during 40s. Females occurs after sixth decades. Males have receding hair especially from parietal and temporal areas. The age of onset, extent and rate of hair loss varies from person to person.

PATHOGENESIS

Testosterone is converted to dihydrotestosterone and increase in dihydrotestisterone causes balding.

Laboratory Investigations

Trichogram: Increase of percentage of telogen hairs.
Hormone testosterone, dihydroepiandrosterone sulphate, prolactin, serum iron, ferritin, skin biopsy.

Management

Finestride: 1 mg daily inhibits conversion of testosterone to dihydrotestosterone. It lowers scalp level of dihydrotestosterone.

Surgical Treatment

Grafts of follicles are taken from androgen insensitive hair sites, peripheral occipital and parietal hairy areas to bald androgen sensitive areas. These could be treated by scalp reduction and rotation flaps.

Hair transplantation is surgical technique where individual hair follicles are transplanted. Hair transplant procedure called follicular unit transplantation. Follicular unit transplantation where individual follicles of hair are removed are between 0.6 and 1.25 mm diameter. Each follicle is reinserted using a microblade. Recovery is within 7 days. Excised strip is 1–1.5 × 15–30 cm in size. Long sessions are required for follicular unit extraction. The hair follicles is complex structure containing cell types that produce special proteins. These proteins govern the continuous cycling of follicles through its stages of anagen, catagen, telagen, and exogen. Hair transplantation is mainstay of hair restoration. New methods for delivering molecules to follicles is by gene therapy. Walter Unger defined the parameters of safe donor zone from which permanent hair follicles could be extracted for hair transplantation. He described the identification of follicular unit and elucidation of its role on follicular techniques.[1] Hair follicle regeneration from follicular fragments and dissociated cells. Trichogenic culture and delivery into patients are future horizons for hair restoration.[2]

Tissue expansion is ideally suited for expansion of hair bearing skin of scalp if hair has been lost through trauma or disease. Surgical tissue expander is expandable balloon constructed of silicon with means of introducing fluids placed beneath skin adjacent to defect. Volume injected depends on site, discomfort and anticipated expansion. Tissue is technique of gaining extra skin by subcutaneous insertion of silicon which could be expanded by injection of saline over several weeks to cover large scalp defects.

Excessive hair is common cosmetic problem. Congenital adrenal hyperplasia, polycystic ovary, hirsutism, hypertrichosis are common conditions causing it. Methods of hair excision are shaving and depilation. Thioglycolates are used to disrupt disulphide bridges. Epilation is removal of entire shaft. Waxing is one of the effective methods which lasts for several weeks. Threading is practiced by cosmetologists. Electrolysis is insertion of fine needles into follicles to damage it. Temporary reduction of hair is by eflornithine hydrochloride cream applied which inhibits ornithine decarboxylase.

LASERS

Light amplification by stimulated emission of radiation. Clinical conditions treated by lasers

Skin resurfacing	– CO_2, erbium-YAG laser
Pigmented lesions	– Nd:YAG laser
Tattoos	– Nd:YAG laser
Hair excision	– Long pulsed diode
Vascular lesions	– Pulsed dye laser

Laser hair removal is by destroying pleuripotent cells by heat conducted from melanin of follicle.

Types of Laser System for Hair Excision

Long pulsed 694 nm
Long pulsed alexandrite 755 nm
Long pulsed diode laser 810 nm
Long pulsed Nd:YAG laser 1064 nm
Intense pulsed light 500–1200 nm
Longer wavelengths are used for better skin penetration. Nd:YAG is better for darker skins.

References

1. Unger WP. Delineating the safe donor for hair transplantation. Am J Cosmetic Surg 1994;11:239–43.

2. Marshell BT, Ingraham CA, Wiu X, et al. New potential cell sources of hair restoration. Facial Plast Clin North Am 2013;21(3): 521–8.

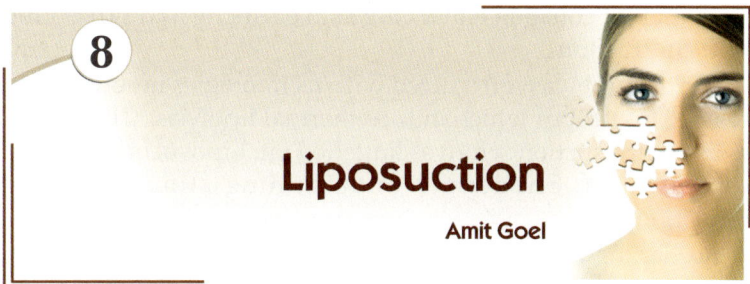

Liposuction

Amit Goel

Liposuction is the most common cosmetic procedure in the USA. Most plastic surgeons perform suction assisted ultrasound assisted and power assisted lipoaspirate. Liposuction refered as liposculpture is form of surgical body contouring that aims to reduce focal subcutaneous, suprafacial fat accumulation at different sites by transcutaneous vacuum assisted extraction of fat particles through small punctures in skin. Liposuction was introduced in 1976 by Fischer who pioneered use of hollow cannula.

Illouz refined the process of liposuction and their contributions including wet techniques, injection of hypotonic saline and hyaluronic acid.[1] Liposuction removes fat through small incisions with atraumatic cannulas. Liposuction was developed for removal of fat from abdomen and subcutaneous tissue. Liposuction causes volume reduction and body reshaping. Lipoplasty is similar to liposuction only that fat is removed differentially from different areas. Common areas are abdomen, buttoks, thighs, hips, arms, breast, chin and face. In males 60% fats lies in subcutaneous plane and external fat removal makes body lighter. In hips, thighs, buttocks fat lies in subcutaneous plane and external fat removal makes body lighter.

Abdominal liposuction is started beneath breast. Suction assisted liposuction was preferred method of fat removal for 51.4%. Laser liposuction is recent innovation in lipossculpture. Advantages are reduced bruising, edema and early recovery. Laser liposuction is based on thermal effect. Laser stimulates formation of collagen enhancing skin elasticity and promoting skin contraction.

Ultrasound was introduced with technologies involving use of laser tip probes which induce thermal lipolysis. Ultrasound assisted liposuction removes liquefied fat. Liposuction cannula aspirates fat. Subdermal undermining stimulates skin retraction.

Reshaping abdomen involves excision of abdomen and fat and tightening of rectus abdominis muscle. Goal of skin excision is to remove the skin between umbilicus and pubis. The abdominal skin and fat are elevated from underlying musculature. Abdominal muscles are invaginated and laxity removed by sutures. Umbilicus is repositioned after skin excision.

PROCEDURE

Patient draped and after local anaesthesia puncture is made and blunt tipped infusion cannula is inserted and infusion of tumescent fluid is done. Cannula is advanced and several areas of fat, subdermal, mid and deeper fat should be infused and suctioned. Common infusion rates less than 100 ml/min. Continual manipulation of skin and subcutaneous tissue is neceessary for appropriate amounts of fat to be removed. Subcutaneous infiltration is done to facilitate adipolysis and aspiration. Suction assisted liposuction causes mechanical disruption. Postoperative compression are required for 6–8 weeks. Lateral hips, legs, and abdomen are common sites for liposuction.

Literature

Dr Jeffrey Klein in 1985 introduced microcannular tumescent liposuction which made liposuction safer and became safe and day care surgery. He introduced 3.5 mm cannulae for extraction. Safe limit of fat removed is 5 litres.[2]

The safety and efficacy has established this technique the gold standard method of liposuction.[3]

A major application of this technique has been for management of gynaecomastia. Recent advances include laser lipolysis and ultrasound lipolysis. For any cosmetic procedure including liposuction, safe and satisfactory result is more important than quick results.[4]

Hanke et al studied 15336 cases of liposuction performed by members of American dermatological surgery. They found minor complications.[5] A survey was carried by 517 dermatological surgeons, members of dermatological surgery in august 2001 for cases between 1994 and 2000. Based on this study of 66570 cases complications were 0.68 per 1000 cases. Data from 26259 patients who had undergone liposuction was collected and incidence of postoperative pain, fibrosis was similar in different liposuction techniques.[6] Liposuction removes fat through small incisions with atraumatic cannulas. Laser lipolysis is based on thermal effect. Laser lipolysis stimulates formation of collagen enhancing skin elasticity and promoting skin contraction.[7]

Suction assisted liposuction is preferred method of fat removal for 51.4%. Ultrasound assisted liposuction and laser assisted liposuction had complications.[8] Laser lipolysis is recent technique in liposculpture. Advantages are reduced bruising, edema, pain and early recovery.[9] Lipoabdominoplasty is technique to contour the abdomen and flanks. 1316 lipo-abdominoplasty patients were studied and lipoaspirate was 1605 ml, weight of resected tissue 1039 g and time 225 minutes, it was safe and effective procedure.[10]

References

1. Illouz YG. Body contouring by lipolysis 5 year experience with 3000 cases. Plast Reconst surg 1983;72:591–7.

2. Klin JA, The Tumescent technique for liposuction surgery. J Am acad cosmet surg 1987;4:263–7.

3. Ostad A, Kageyama N, Moy RL. Tumescent anesthesis with a lidocaine dose of 55 mg/kg is safe for liposuction. Dermatol Surg 1996;22;921–7.

4. Nahi FR, Nahai F. MOC-PSSM, CME article. Plast Reconst Surg 2008;121(1).

5. Hanke CW, Burnstein G, Bullock S. Safety of tumescent liposuction in 15336 patients. National survey results. Dermatol Surg 1995; 21:459–62.

6. Houseman TS, Lawrence N, Mellen BG. The safety of liposuction, results of a national survey. Dermatol Surg 2002;28:971–8.

7. Triana L, Triana C, Barbato C, et al. Liposuction 25 year experience in 26259 patients using different devices. Aesthetic Surg 2009: Nov–Dec; 29(6):509–12.

8. Mordon S, Plot E. Laser lipolysis vs traditional liposuction for fat removal. Expert rev meddevices 2009 Nov; (6):677–88.

9. Ahmad J, Eaves FF, Rohrich RJ, et al. The American society of aesthetic plastic surg survey, current trends in liposuction. Aesthet Surg J 2011 Feb; 31(2):214–24.

10. Levesque AY, Daniels MA, Polynice A. Outpatient lipoabdomino-plasty; review of literature and practical considerations of safe practice, Aesthet Surg J 2013 Sep 1;33(7):1021–9.

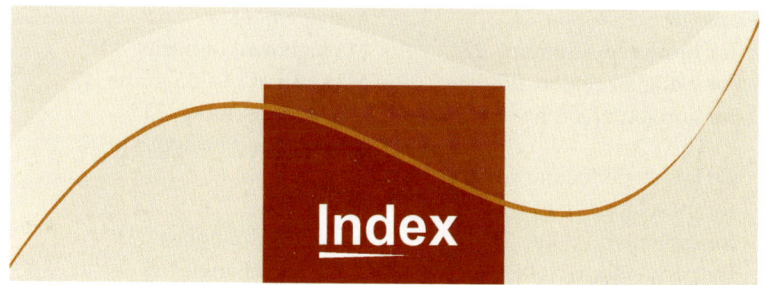

Index